EDWARD T. HECK, Ph.D., is Assistant Director of Research and Project Director, Boston Children's Service Association. ANGEL G. GOMEZ, M.D., is Director of Community Psychiatry and Forensic Psychiatry, the Puerto Rico Institute of Psychiatry. GEORGE L. ADAMS, M.D., is Special Assistant to the Director, National Institute of Mental Health.

D1399911

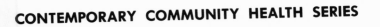
CONTEMPORARY COMMUNITY HEALTH SERIES

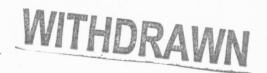

A GUIDE TO MENTAL HEALTH SERVICES

A GUIDE
TO

Edward T. Heck, Ph.D.
Angel G. Gomez, M.D.
George L. Adams, M.D.

MENTAL HEALTH
SERVICES

University of Pittsburgh Press

Publication of this book was made possible by a grant from the Maurice Falk Medical Fund. The Fund, however, is not the author, publisher, or proprietor of the material presented here and is not to be understood, by virtue of its grant, as endorsing any statement made or expressed herein.

Library of Congress Cataloging in Publication Data

Heck, Edward T.   date
  A guide to mental health services.

  (Contemporary community health series)
  Includes bibliographical references.
  1. Community mental health services. I. Gomez, Angel G., date   joint author. II. Adams, George L., date   joint author.   III. Title.   IV. Series. [DNLM: 1. Community mental health services—U.S. 2. Mental health services—U.S. WM30 H448g 1973]
RA790.H42   362.2'097   72-92694
ISBN 0-8229-3262-8
ISBN 0-8229-5236-X (pbk.)

Publication of this book
was made possible by a grant
from the Maurice Falk Medical Fund.

To Martha, Joffin, and Josie

Contents

Preface

The purpose of this book is to present basic, comprehensive, and useful information about mental health services, practitioners, and treatments that will enable the reader to become a better-informed and more discriminating user of mental health services.

Patients or clients of practitioners, clinics, and hospitals are the most obvious consumers of mental health services. Their ability to procure satisfactory services from the mental health service system depends upon a knowledge of this complex system and an understanding of the relationships between its various parts. Unfortunately, many people need to enter the mental health service system at the height of some crisis. They may, for example, be disoriented or experiencing severe stress, or they may be abandoned or abused children. The success of these people in obtaining timely and appropriate treatment often depends solely upon the knowledge, experience, and judgment of others who assume the responsibility of guiding them into and through this complex human service system. These guides are the people who help those with mental problems to obtain appropriate assistance when they need it. It is for these guides that this book is written.

Although "mental health" is something that nearly everyone is concerned about, it is an issue about which no one seems to know very much. Despite what amounts to a national preoccupation with matters related to psychiatry and psychology, too few people appear to know a great deal about mental health practitioners and what they do, or about the agencies and institutions in which they do it. Two factors are major contributors to the widespread lack of useful public information about mental health issues. These are the "look the other way" attitudes that have been developed about mental disorders over the years, and the vague and mysterious language used by those who seem to be experts in the field. Although few professional areas are characterized by as little a degree of internal consensus as the field of mental health, still there would probably be general agreement among its professionals on one point: there is a marked sellers' market favoring the providers over the consumers of mental health services.

Clearly the consumer and those responsible for guiding him to the procurement of satisfactory mental health services need more than interest in order to make efficient use of the vast network of mental health services existing today. They need a body of basic, understandable, and integrated facts about the problems, practitioners, diagnostic and treatment techniques, and settings where the various mental health professionals practice their specialties. With such information they would know how to approach a mental health agency appropriately, and what realistically to expect of it when the potential client arrives there. But most important, those guiding the client would be in a position to represent his interests by asking specific and answerable questions about the services offered and the financial and emotional costs that might be involved in accepting them. Also, if certain prescribed procedures seemed unclear or ill advised they could intelligently ask for clarification or alternatives. Finally, if they were still not satisfied with the services, they would be aware of some possibilities for correcting the situation either by obtaining other professional consultation or by going through legal, political, or community action channels.

A Guide to Mental Health Services is intended to provide the reader with a compilation of information about a broad range of mental health topics. It is not meant to be a directory of services, but a key that we hope the reader will find useful as he begins to search out and evaluate the mental health services in his local community.

Acknowledgments

This book was written while the authors were postdoctoral fellows at the Laboratory of Community Psychiatry, Harvard Medical School. Our colleagues, Dr. Thomas Bigham, Dr. Anthony Broskowski, Dr. Barbara Clemence, Dr. Stephen Creel, Prof. Anne Hargreaves, Dr. Melva Jo Hendrix, Dr. Harold Jarmon, Dr. Peter Johnston, Dr. James Kelz, Dr. Farrokh Khajavi, Dr. Dubravkc Kuftinec, Dr. William Mermis, and Dr. Joan Ward Mullaney, influenced our thinking, our practice, and the contents of this book. We would also like to acknowledge the influence of the many dedicated teachers under whom we have been privileged to study and learn.

Mrs. Diane Nicholls was a great help to us in editing the first draft of the manuscript. We are especially grateful to Mrs. Evelyn Stone for her interest, advice, and editorial assistance in the presentation and preparation of the manuscript for publication.

The content of this book is the sole responsibility of the authors and in no way reflects upon the Laboratory of Community Psychiatry, the Massachusetts Department of Mental Health, the Puerto Rico Institute of Psychiatry, or the National Institute of Mental Health.

A GUIDE TO MENTAL HEALTH SERVICES

El respeto al derecho ajeno es la paz.
(Respect for the rights of others is the essence of peace.)

Benito Juarez

CHAPTER 1

Mental Health and Mental Illness

Mental Health

Both *mental* and *health* are extremely complex concepts; taken separately, each has been the subject of several hundred scholarly books. When they are combined to form the term *mental health*, the result is an even more complex concept that has, in turn, stimulated more scholarly works and seemingly endless debate and discussion. This particular aspect of the current information explosion places the potential consumer of mental health services at a decided disadvantage because he cannot possibly expect to locate, effectively utilize, and critically evaluate the services he needs *unless* he can speak and understand the expanding mental health "language."

We will begin by defining a *concept* as a formulation about the way in which some events or objects are ordered. A concept is an idea, or a kind of mental shorthand. Health, for example, is an idea about the condition a person is in. You cannot "see" health (since it is a concept), but you *can* see some signs which lead you to believe that the person you are observing is in a state of good health.

In order to gain a working knowledge of the concept of mental health, we will examine the two components *mental* and *health* separately, starting with the latter.

Health as a Concept

There are two ways of conceptualizing health, one *ideal* and the other *operational*. As an ideal concept, health can be defined as a state of general well-being. This is an ideal concept because it refers to an ideal and positively desirable state. Unfortunately, only a small fraction of people are ideally healthy. For organizational planning purposes (e.g., establishing national priorities), ideal health is a worthwhile and useful concept because it calls attention to the necessity for promoting health. An individual in need of a particular service, however, will find an operational (or working) definition of health more useful. Thus health can be operationally defined as the absence of illness. According to this operational definition, a "sick" person who submits to some particular health service can be considered cured (or restored to health) when he is no longer "sick." Throughout this book the concept health will always be used in the operational sense unless it is clearly noted otherwise.

Since the concept health refers to the state a person is in or to the level at which he is functioning, we might easily break down the concept further by specifying the various states he might be in or the various ways in which he might be functioning. For example, we frequently describe general areas of a person's functioning by referring to his physical health, mental health, emotional health, spiritual health, and so on. Human beings can function in any number of ways and can therefore be said to be healthy in any number of ways. Although all of these ways of functioning are related to one another in a given individual, it is quite possible for a person to be physically healthy but mentally unhealthy, or vice versa, at the same time.

Combining Mental *with* Health

The concept *mental* refers to a general area of human functioning, that is, the broad area of functioning that includes the several human activities related to the working of the brain and the nervous system. But we frequently discuss mental functioning by breaking it down into smaller, more precise units. Thus, we often include specific mental activities such as intellectual functioning, emotional functioning, or social functioning under the general heading "mental functioning." When the two concepts *mental* and *health* are combined they refer both to a general *area* of functioning (mental) and to a general *level* of functioning (health).

In the ideal sense, the promotion of mental health, or a state of general mental well-being, is the responsibility of various units of society like the family, schools, and the government. Professional persons working in the field of mental health can only assist in the achievement of this goal by pointing out ways in which general mental well-being might be promoted in the population and by formulating appropriate long-range plans for its achievement.

Most mental health professionals are not large-scale public planners but, rather, trained workers who try to remedy currently existing mental problems for individuals. The consumer of mental health services will most likely encounter these professionals working as technicians who apply their skills to the solution of a particular problem. In this capacity they usually function best as systems analysts, troubleshooters, or problem solvers for individuals and/or relatively small groups of people. The kinds of problems to which they apply their time and talents are variously called "mental illness," "interpersonal disorders," or "emotional disturbances," to name but a few. And these terms introduce another instance of language confusion and quite naturally lead us to the next step in learning about the mental health language.

Mental Illness

Illness is a concept that refers to a specific impairment in some area of a person's functioning. In common usage, the term illness refers primarily to a person's physical condition. In the context of mental health, however, illness has a much broader meaning, including all those areas of human functioning which are related to the working of the brain and the nervous system. In the ideal sense, illness refers to any state of functioning other than ideal health. In the operational sense the term refers to the existence of an impairment of the normal functioning in some area of a person's mental activity. Because there are so many possible ways of describing areas of mental functioning, there are a correspondingly large number of ways of referring to functional impairments. For example, we frequently refer to "emotional disturbances," "psychological disorders," and "interpersonal problems" under the general heading of "mental illness," provided, of course, that the particular malfunction we are describing is serious enough to represent a genuine impairment of that specific area of mental activity. For the purposes of this book we will consider such terms as *illness, prob-*

lem, and *disorder,* which refer to a serious impairment of some area of mental functioning, as being roughly synonymous, even though each implies different levels or amounts of impairment. And unless it is clearly stipulated otherwise, these terms will be used in the operational sense throughout the book.

In the mental health sense both health and illness are relative terms. Thus, one must have some standard in order to judge how well or how poorly a person is functioning. For example, imagine that a social worker on duty at the emergency service of a community mental health center receives a call from a distraught person who relates that he has just observed a girl in the public park smearing ice cream in her hair and babbling incoherently. One of the first things the social worker would want to know is the age of the girl. If the caller estimates the girl's age at sixteen or seventeen years, the social worker would have good reason to suspect that the girl in the park has a legitimate mental disorder since the behavior reported by the caller is highly unusual for a girl of that age. If, on the other hand, the caller estimates the girl's age to be about two years, the social worker would probably not be concerned since the behavior reported by the caller is not at all unusual for a two-year-old child. It is also safe to say that in the latter case, the alert social worker would immediately focus his professional attention on the distraught caller. But that is another story.

In this fictitious example the standard against which the level of functioning was measured was age-appropriate behavior. Every culture, ours included, has developed a complex set of standards for making the distinction between normal and abnormal functioning, and these factors must be considered in any judgment about the "normality" or "abnormality" of a particular person's mental functioning. Thus, whereas the shrinking of heads might indicate a high level of socially accepted competence in some parts of Borneo, the same practice would be considered highly bizarre and deviant if it were attempted in Boston.

An accurate professional diagnosis is an extremely complex statement. It would have to consider a number of important factors such as the seriousness of the disability as the afflicted person experiences it, the person's available resources for rectifying the problem, and the situational factors which may be related to the problem. In order to con-

sider an individual's behavior as a "mental problem," the absolute minimum information one has to have is (1) what *area* of mental functioning
is involved and (2) *how* serious the impairment is. Of the many complex factors that have to be considered in the actual diagnosis of a mental problem, these two should always be the starting point. We can consider as a working guideline the possibility that a person has a mental
problem if some particular area of his mental functioning is impaired to
the point that it directly and seriously causes discomfort to himself or
others.

Diagnostic Labels and Their Uses

Broadly speaking, a diagnosis is a description of a mental problem.
In some cases the problem is described in considerable detail, with men-
tion made of the area of functioning that is impaired, the level or seriousness of the impairment, the conditions under which it occurs, how
often it occurs, and how long the impairment has been in existence.
This kind of detailed description, or diagnosis, is sometimes called a
functional description of the mental problem. Ideally, such descriptions
should be understandable, orderly, and useful.

Another way of describing mental problems is to group certain disorders that have something in common and to refer to them by the
group heading, or diagnostic label. A diagnostic label is a kind of shorthand used by mental health professionals for referring to a particular
problem as a member of a group of problems that (presumably) have
something in common. For example, different mental problems might
be labeled "psychotic," "neurotic," "schizophrenic," or "phobic." The
lack of specific and detailed information in these labels might be toler-
able *if* everyone who used them were in agreement as to precisely what
they meant. Unfortunately, however, there is widespread ambiguity and
lack of agreement surrounding the use of these labels both within the
mental health professions and within the population in general. This
situation has grown progressively worse as psychiatric jargon has become incorporated into everyday language.

Diagnostic labels might be used advantageously in certain specific and
limited situations. Examples of such circumstances might be those in

which professional colleagues are in agreement as to the precise meaning of the labels, or in which such a label is required for record purposes as a qualification for a pension or a disability benefit.

On the other hand, there are many sound reasons for not using diagnostic labels. An important case in point is the defensive position in which the consumer of mental health services finds himself when these terms are used to describe his condition or his situation. For example, consider the fact that when a diagnostic label is used to describe a patient's problem, it is commonly said that he *is* neurotic or psychotic or compulsive or whatever. Notice that, as if by magic, the label has expanded to cover what the patient *is* (as opposed to what the patient *does*). Instead of being a functional description of a specific mental impairment, the diagnostic label serves as an ambiguous and pejorative statement about the patient's whole personality.

If one hears or reads of a patient's being referred to by means of a diagnostic label, one should immediately demand clarification in the form of a functional description of the problem in understandable, orderly, and useful language. In accordance with this advice, an attempt will be made throughout this book to refrain from using diagnostic labels.

CHAPTER 2

Some Mental Health Professions

This chapter will introduce three important professional groups that work in the area of mental health: psychiatrists, psychologists, and social workers. These groups in particular have been chosen for discussion because (1) they are the professional groups most likely to be encountered by the average person in need of the widest variety of mental health services, and (2) members of these three groups work together in almost every kind of mental health facility. The term *profession* is used here to mean a body of persons who are qualified to practice a vocation or occupation requiring advanced training in some formal discipline; and each of the three professional groups will be examined in terms of this definition.

One will undoubtedly notice the amount of duplication in the professional activities that these groups provide. This partial overlapping may be due in part to the fact that the official definitions of these three professional roles are noticeably nonspecific. There is, however, a great deal of variation not only in the activities of the individual professional groups, but also in the requirements for practice from state to state and even from agency to agency. With the exception of prescribing drugs and administering certain medical treatments, there appears to be very little "mental health" activity that is the exclusive province of any of the professions operating in the field. Each profession's definition of itself and of its activities will be given in this chapter as a kind of background, but a list of publications and other information sources is given in chapter 10 for those who may want more detailed information about any of the topics dealt with in this chapter.

Psychiatry

Definition of a Psychiatrist

A psychiatrist is a *physician* who specializes in the diagnosis and treatment of mental disorders.[1] Any licensed physician can practice psychiatry in the same way that he is free to practice any of the other medical specialties, such as surgery or obstetrics. The psychiatrist has become a specialist by virtue of his advanced training and experience in the area of psychiatry, the branch of medicine that deals with the causes, diagnosis, treatment, and prevention of mental and emotional disorders. It is also concerned with mental retardation.

Basic Qualifications

In order to become a psychiatrist, a person must meet the following requirements:

1. He must have earned a Doctor of Medicine (M.D.) or Doctor of Osteopathy (D.O.) degree.
2. He must have successfully completed an approved, three-year residency training program in psychiatry.[2]
3. He must be licensed as a physician in the state where he is practicing. An unrestricted license as a physician would permit the psychiatrist to practice privately if he desired to do so. Also issued are restricted medical licenses, which would permit the psychiatrist to practice only in certain settings like mental hospitals, university clinics, and correctional institutions.

Board-certified Psychiatrists

The American Board of Psychiatry and Neurology is a private, nonprofit corporation whose purpose is to maintain high standards in the practice of the medical specialties of psychiatry and neurology. This control is held by issuing certificates or diplomas to those physicians

---

1. L. E. Hinsie and R. J. Campbell, *Psychiatric Dictionary*, 3rd ed. (New York: Oxford University Press, 1960), p. 604.

2. The American Board of Psychiatry and Neurology, Inc. recently eliminated the completion of the internship as a requirement for certification by the Board.

who meet the rigorous requirements for certification by the Board. In order to be certified by the Board, a psychiatrist must meet the following requirements:

1. He must have successfully completed a three-year-residency training program approved by the Board.
2. He must have completed an additional two years of practice following completion of the residency training program.
3. He must have passed a rigorous set of written and oral examinations in psychiatry.

Some Subspecialties of Psychiatry

Because of the broad scope and complexities of psychiatry, many psychiatrists specialize, focusing their professional activities on a specific population or a particular subarea of the overall specialty of psychiatry. These subareas exist because some abnormalities of the physical and personality growth processes are prevalent in certain age groups, occupational groups, and the like. A psychiatrist's personal preference for and commitment to a special area in psychiatry is strongly influenced by his own personality and interests.

General psychiatry. The general psychiatrist deals mainly with the mental disorders of adulthood, but many concern themselves as well with the mental problems of families and children.

Child psychiatry. Child psychiatrists are involved particularly with disorders of infancy, childhood, and adolescence. In addition to the other skills he must develop, the child psychiatrist must master the delicate art of communicating with children and young people. Because child psychiatry is itself a very broad area of study and practice, there is some interest today in separating this subspecialty into two subspecialties: child psychiatry and adolescent psychiatry.

Geriatric psychiatry. Geriatric psychiatrists concentrate their professional activities on behavioral problems resulting from the process of advanced aging: they work with problematic behaviors caused by organic brain conditions as well as with mental problems of older people that result from their being retired, widowed, incapacitated, and so forth.

Industrial psychiatry. Industrial psychiatrists deal with the prevention, diagnosis, and treatment of mental and emotional disorders arising within the areas of work and employment.

Military psychiatry. Military psychiatrists apply the specialty of general psychiatry to military life and to the mental problems found arising within it.

Administrative psychiatry. Administrative psychiatrists specialize in handling the complex problems of managing institutions and facilities that diagnose and treat mental disorders. They deal with both hospital administration (requiring special certification) and administrative procedures regarding programs in other mental health settings.

Forensic psychiatry. Forensic psychiatrists focus most of their time and attention on people who may or may not show evidence of mental disorders and have come to the attention of the law. "The forensic psychiatrist must have a practical working knowledge of the law, not only in the judicial aspect of the criminal, civil, and appellate areas, but also in the legislative aspects, for it is through legislation that law and psychiatry can cooperate in forming practical and workable approaches to the problems of the mentally ill participant in a legal proceeding."[3] (See also "Adult Offenders: Services Through the Courts" in chapter 9.)

Community psychiatry. Community psychiatrists deal with the diagnosis, treatment, and prevention of mental disorders on a community-wide basis. Community psychiatry is not a formal subspecialty of psychiatry, but refers instead to the type of professional activity of a group of psychiatrists. Community psychiatrists are most often found directing community mental health centers, working in various agencies and institutes of the government, serving as consultants to various mental health programs, and teaching in universities. They provide direct service to patients and help other care givers mainly through consultation and training.

In some places industrial psychiatry, forensic psychiatry, and religion and psychiatry are covered by the term community psychiatry.

3. A. Robey and W. J. Bogard, "The Compleat Forensic Psychiatrist," *American Journal of Psychiatry* 126, no. 4 (October 1969): 525.

Requirements for Independent Practice

Mandatory. The practitioner of psychiatry must be currently licensed as a physician in the state in which he is practicing.

Optional. The practitioner of psychiatry may be certified by the American Board of Psychiatry and Neurology.

Psychology

Definition of a Psychologist

A psychologist is a person who has earned an advanced university degree in psychology, the science of behavior. In addition to possessing either a master's degree (M.A.) or a doctoral degree (Ph.D.), certain subspecialties of applied psychology require additional periods of training and/or supervised experience.

It should be noted that several states have license or registration requirements for psychologists which restrict the title "psychologist" to those persons who have earned the doctoral degree. Under these regulations persons holding the master's degree are classified as "psychological examiners," "school diagnosticians," or by some term other than "psychologist."

Basic Qualifications

There is no universally accepted set of criteria applicable to all psychologists in all states, but there are five areas which may generally be used as measures of the level of qualification of psychologists. These five rules are:

1. Academic: the earning of formal university degrees (M.A., Ph.D., Ed.D., etc.)
2. The completion of certain supervised experiences, like clinical or school internships
3. Membership status in professional associations, primarily the American Psychological Association and the various state psychological associations

4. Licensing, certification, or registration of psychologists imposed and enforced by state governments

5. Possession of a diploma issued by the American Board of Professional Psychology (ABPP)

Licensing and Certification

Two levels of state regulation of professional services are licensing and certification. A *license* is "permission, granted according to legal provisions, to practice a profession or occupation. In general, the term is not used unless the occupation is forbidden to those without a license."[4] *Certification* is "a statement by an official body that a person or institution has complied with or met certain standards of excellence. . . . Under compulsory certification for psychologists, no person may represent himself to be a psychologist unless certified by a legally established board. This does not, however, limit psychological practice to those certified. When practice is restricted, licensure is the proper term."[5]

Knowledge of the licensing and certification requirements for psychologists in the various states is important for two reasons. First, the level of professional regulation imposed upon practitioners by the state offers the consumer some standardized information about providers of these services in his locality. Second, the level of professional regulation imposed by the state affords a clue about how active and demanding it is likely to be in intervening in disputes that may arise between consumers and providers of regulated services. Table 1 shows the particular forms of regulation to be found in the American states and various Canadian provinces.

Diplomates of the American Board of Professional Psychology

The American Board of Professional Psychology encourages the pursuit of excellence in professional psychology by issuing and controlling diplomas that recognize the highest level of professional competence (as judged by professional peers). Application for diplomas is purely volun-

4. H. B. English and A. C. English, *A Comprehensive Dictionary of Psychological and Psychoanalytical Terms* (New York: David McKay Co., 1958), p. 295.

5. Ibid., p. 82.

Table 1

REGULATION OF PSYCHOLOGISTS IN AMERICAN STATES AND
CANADIAN PROVINCES

States Having License Laws

Alabama	Idaho	Oklahoma
Alaska	Kentucky	Pennsylvania
Arkansas	Maine	South Carolina
Colorado	Massachusetts	Tennessee
District of Columbia	Montana	Texas
Florida	Nebraska	Virginia
Georgia	New Jersey	West Virginia
Hawaii	North Carolina	Wisconsin
	Ohio	

States and Provinces Having Registration and Certification Acts

Alberta	Manitoba	North Dakota
Arizona	Maryland	Ontario
California	Michigan	Oregon
Connecticut	Minnesota	Quebec
Delaware	Mississippi	Rhode Island
Illinois	Nevada	Saskatchewan
Indiana	New Brunswick	Utah
Kansas	New Hampshire	Washington
Louisiana	New Mexico	Wyoming
	New York	

States and Provinces Having Nonstatutory Certifying Agencies

British Columbia	Missouri	Vermont
Iowa	South Dakota	

SOURCE: *American Psychological Association Directory* (Washington, D.C., 1968).

tary and covers four areas of professional psychological activity: clinical psychology, counseling psychology, industrial and organizational psychology, and school psychology.

Requirements for the ABPP diplomas include:

1. A Ph.D. degree in the appropriate area of psychology
2. At least five years of qualifying experience

3. Membership in the American (or Canadian) Psychological Association
4. Successful completion of written and oral examinations
5. Submission of a detailed work sample
6. A professional reputation of unquestioned integrity and competence

Some Subspecialties of Psychology

Clinical psychology. Clinical psychology is the branch of psychology that deals with the diagnosis and treatment of abnormal behavior by psychological means. Clinical psychologists are perhaps best known for their skillful use of psychological tests. In addition, however, they are highly trained both in psychotherapy and in methods of psychological research.

Counseling psychology. Counseling psychologists deal with specific problems of living that may or may not include mental problems or seriously abnormal behavior. Marriage counseling and vocational counseling are examples of specific life problems handled by counseling psychologists.

Educational and school psychology. Educational and school psychologists focus on problems of learning and socialization in school settings. They often apply their skills to the design of teaching methods and curricula to be used in various areas of the schools. One important aspect of the school psychologist's work involves serving as a consultant or resource person for teachers and school administrators in matters relating to the mental health of the students. In this capacity he is frequently the first professional person to come into contact with a young person experiencing a behavioral or emotional problem.

Community psychology. Community psychologists are involved with the diagnosis, treatment, and prevention of psychological problems on a community-wide basis. For example, a community psychologist might identify an unusually high level of learning disability or behavior disorder in a particular part of a city or in a single school district. He would then devise ways of mobilizing the community's treatment resources to solve those problems and to prevent their occurrence in the future. This activity may include specialized consultation with other mental health professionals or the provision of training and assistance for other groups concerned with mental disorders within the community, such as policemen, clergymen, and schoolteachers.

Requirements for Independent Practice

Mandatory. The independent practitioner of psychology must comply with state licensing laws for psychologists in the state in which he is practicing. He must comply with the provisions of certification acts relative to the use of the title "psychologist" in those states where certification acts are in effect. (See table 1.)

Optional. The American Psychological Association has published the following guidelines for the qualifications of independently practicing psychologists.[6] A psychologist must:

1. have been awarded a diploma by the American Board of Professional Psychology (ABPP), or
2. been licensed or certified by the state governing boards, or
3. been certified by voluntary boards established by the state psychological associations.

Social Work

Definition of a Professional Social Worker

A professional social worker is a person who has earned an MSW, a master's degree in social work, which is a helping profession dealing with a broad range of human problems and social needs. A social worker is often the first professional person a client meets when he brings a problem to a mental health service organization. Social workers often have the responsibility of interviewing prospective clients in order to gather information essential for the solution of mental disorders. Social workers also provide individual and group psychotherapy, assistance in finding homes or employment for persons with special needs, and assistance in organizing groups of people to solve specific problems. Many social workers also occupy executive and administrative positions in mental health programs and facilities.

Basic Qualifications

According to the National Association of Social Workers (NASW), the minimum required standard of professional competence in social work

6. *American Psychological Association Directory* (Washington, D.C., 1968) p. xxxvi.

is membership in the Academy of Certified Social Workers (ACSW).[7] ACSW is a nonstatutory certification system begun by the delegate assembly of NASW in 1960. Requirements for membership in the Academy are:

1. Membership in NASW (which requires a master's degree in social work)
2. Two years of successful social work experience in one agency under the supervision of a member of ACSW
3. Successful completion of a national qualifying examination.

Members of the Academy of Certified Social Workers may use the initials ACSW after their names.

Formal Education

Several universities and colleges which are accredited by the Council on Social Work Education offer professional degrees in social work. The most common degree is Master of Social Work (MSW), which requires about two years of academic work and field experience beyond a bachelor's degree. Some schools offer a Doctor of Social Welfare (DSW) degree or a Doctor of Philosophy (Ph.D.) degree for those desiring additional training. These advanced degrees usually require about three years of study beyond the MSW degree, and most people studying for them would probably be preparing for careers in teaching, research, administration, or advanced practice.

Certification

According to NASW[8] the following ten states and Puerto Rico have some form of regulation: California, Illinois, Louisiana, Maine, New York, Oklahoma, Rhode Island, South Carolina, Utah, and Virginia. One state, California, has a licensing law for clinical social workers as well as a registration law.

---

7. R. Morris, ed., *Encyclopedia of Social Work*, 2 vols., 16th issue (New York: National Association of Social Workers, 1971), 2:1480.
8. National Association of Social Workers, "Information on Legal Regulation of Social Work," mimeographed (New York: 10 August 1972).

Some Fields of Social Work Practice

According to *The Encyclopedia of Social Work* "a field of social work practice centers around some major human need or social problem and is a part of the services organized to meet the need or problem."[9] Social workers are employed in many capacities in mental health service organizations, and the services they provide range from intake screening to aftercare and follow-up. Social workers may also be found working in other organizations related to the mental health service system—schools, courts, and social agencies. Still others may concentrate their professional energies in the delivery of specific services such as group work.

Schools. School social workers frequently provide short-term psychotherapy to students who are experiencing difficulties in school, home, or community. They often facilitate the delivery of social or mental health service by acting as links between the student and the school. In cases where a student or his family requires services not provided by the school system, the school social worker will refer either or both to the appropriate community agency.

Social agency casework. Social agency caseworkers deal with the widest possible range of human activity. In a single day a caseworker may arrange welfare support for a person handicapped by a mental problem, provide marital counseling for a couple facing a domestic crisis, make foster home arrangements for a child when his parent is hospitalized, or coordinate arrangements for a couple who are in the process of adopting an infant.

Group work. Group workers are social workers who have specialized knowledge and training in working with groups of people. These groups are frequently convened in order to solve mental problems being faced by the individual group members. The purpose of the groups may be educational, supportive, organizational, or psychotherapeutic. The group might consist of couples experiencing marital difficulties or, perhaps, adolescents with learning or social problems. In any event, the group's chances of achieving its goals are directly related to the skill of the group leader, who is often a group worker.

9. Morris, *Encyclopedia of Social Work*, 2:1480.

Requirements for Independent Practice

Mandatory. The independent social worker must comply with statutory requirements if he uses the title "social worker" in states where certification acts limit the use of that title. In California he must comply with the licensing law regulating clinical social workers. Those practicing in other areas are not bound by these constraints.[10]

Optional. The National Association of Social Workers (NASW) has published the following guidelines for the qualifications of independently practicing social workers:

1. Graduation from a school of social work accredited by the Council on Social Work Education
2. Membership in NASW
3. Membership in ACSW
4. Five years of acceptable full-time experience in agencies providing supervision by professionally trained social workers, in which two consecutive years were spent in one agency under such supervision while giving direct service and using the method or methods to be used in private practice[11]

Locating a Mental Health Professional Quickly

1. A family physician is in a good position to arrange a timely referral to an appropriate mental health professional.
2. A clergyman, like the family physician, is in a position to make appropriate referrals as well as to provide supportive counsel in times of stress or emergency.
3. The emergency room of a local hospital can refer persons to mental health professionals both on the hospital's staff and practicing in the community.
4. If in the community there is an active community mental health center, it will have a wide range of mental health services, usually available twenty-four hours per day. Emergency (telephone) "hot lines" and "walk-in" clinics are examples of these services.

10. National Association of Social Workers, "Information on Legal Regulation of Social Work."
11. Morris, *Encyclopedia of Social Work,* 2:1480.

5. Local police departments, sheriff's departments, and the state police are vitally important sources of both information and, if necessary, direct assistance in mental health emergencies.
6. Local Visiting Nurse Association offices or public health offices can frequently make appropriate mental health referrals.
7. Telephone directory listings of practitioners and agencies are sometimes useful in emergency situations although they are often not a complete representation of the mental health resources within the community. It is preferable, if the telephone is the only immediately available resource, to ask for assistance from the operator.

Mental Health Professionals: Some Sources of Information

More specific information about the mental health professionals in a particular community may be obtained from the following sources:

1. A community mental health center should be able to provide both printed information and staff assistance in researching the various mental health resources existing within the community.
2. Local mental health agencies, clinics, and hospitals should also be able to furnish information about mental health professionals. The libraries in these facilities ought to contain a good, up-to-date selection of professional association directories.
3. Public libraries usually contain current directories of major professional associations (see chapter 10). State and local chapters of these professional associations may also publish directories, which are usually available in a public library.
4. If copies of these directories are not available in the public library, they can be obtained from the County Health Office, social agencies (like Family Service or Catholic Social Services), the medical library of a hospital, or through a city or county welfare office.
5. The State Department of Licensing and Regulation publishes annual directories of practitioners licensed or certified in a particular state.
6. Direct inquiries can be made to any of the major professional associations, governmental units, or special-interest groups listed in chapter 10.

CHAPTER 3

Diagnosis: Defining Mental Problems

The Diagnostic Process

Diagnosis is the process of identifying, that is, defining and classifying, a health problem. In the mental health context, it involves a professional person's making a formal evaluation of the behavior of his client. Although judgments made by human beings about other humans are never totally without bias, not all biases are bad. We could, in fact, argue that professional training is really a complex set of carefully cultivated biases. What we need to remember at this point is that whenever one person makes a judgment about another, that judgment is influenced to some extent by the past experiences of the person doing the judging.

All human behavior, whether it is grossly deviant or absolutely normative, is the result of a complex set of factors. And most mental health professionals would probably agree that biological, developmental, psychological, and sociocultural factors all exert important influences upon virtually all human behavior. To understand how the different parts of the diagnostic process relate to one another, one could look at the three groups of mental health professionals (psychiatrists, psychologists, and social workers) and see how they function together in the diagnostic process. For purposes of this exercise let us assume that a psychiatrist, a psychologist, and a social worker are working together as a team in the intake section of a mental health clinic.

The task of this mental health team is to investigate all aspects of a behavior problem presented to them by a potential client. They must determine if, in fact, the situation being presented is a legitimate problem. If it is, the team tries to discover the problem's characteristics and boundaries to determine what can be done to solve it. All but the last step, the solution of the problem, are parts of the diagnostic process.

The psychiatrist, being a physician, concerns himself in particular with physical-biological factors. He is careful to note if the client is malnourished, tired, or perhaps intoxicated with either drugs or alcohol. He looks for signs of nervous-system or glandular malfunctioning. He pays particular attention to items in the client's medical history that might provide clues about physical determinants of the present behavior problem. Diseases of the client's parents or relatives or the existence of childhood disease or trauma might provide important clues that the psychiatrist will weigh in arriving at the diagnosis.

The psychologist concentrates on the intellectual, occupational, and social skills of the client. He compares various aspects of the client's functioning in these areas to the functioning of other people who are like the client in many ways—for example, similarity in age and educational level. He attempts to catalogue the client's social and intellectual strengths as well as his weaknesses so that his assets may be incorporated to good advantage into a plan of treatment or rehabilitation.

The objective of the social worker is to gather information about the social network in which the client lives. Family, work, and social relationships are studied in detail, so that all the resources and strengths in the client's environment may be utilized to the fullest in the formulation and execution of the treatment plan.

The point we wish to make with these examples is simply this: most responsible mental health professionals prefer to view their clients as complex human beings whose behavior (both problematic and otherwise) is determined by multiple factors. Consequently, when they are called upon to diagnose a problem, they must gather a lot of information both from the client and from those with whom the client lives and works.

If the client needs help immediately, it may seem irritating to him to be asked dozens of apparently repetitious and irrelevant questions. Questions about whether his mother had diabetes, how well he solves visual organization problems with little blocks, or how many jobs he has had in the last two years may seem to him like a waste of time, but they all are important parts of the diagnostic process. It is also important to realize that the diagnostic activities of the various mental health professionals do not take place in the orderly sequence outlined here. Instead, they may consist of a series of meetings and appointments with various mental health professionals and with other professional persons as well. When involved in a diagnostic process, the mental health professional is really systematically gathering the pieces of a complicated puzzle. His purpose is to gain an understanding of his client as a functioning, complete biological and sociocultural being.

When a person consults a mental health professional in order to solve some problem, it is quite natural that the client's attention will be focused upon the problem which he sees as very troublesome and in need of immediate solution. The mental health professional knows that the client not only has a lot of information about the problem, but also has a wealth of information useful for possible solutions. His task, then, is to find out as much as possible about the presented problem, the client, and the world in which he lives and to organize this material in a way that will lead to a solution of the client's problem.

Let us now examine some specific mental health diagnostic activities.

The Initial Step: The Interview

An interview is a face-to-face meeting for the purpose of conferring about something. In a mental health context, it is a meeting between a professional person and a potential client for the purpose of exchanging information about a problem that the client brings to the practitioner. In the diagnostic phase, this process favors the practitioner, as he is the recipient of more information than he is giving. In the therapeutic phase the balance will shift progressively toward the client, since he receives more information in that phase.

The purpose of a mental health interview is to allow the professional to compile information. The time required for this procedure varies greatly, depending upon the complexity of the problem, the availability of professional resources, the individual work style of the practitioner, and so forth. But it usually requires a series of interviews spread perhaps over a two- or three-week period. The administrative reality of most agency and clinic settings will require a thirty- to sixty-minute period for each interview. Although interviews usually take place in an office or examining room, it is not at all unusual for them to be conducted in the client's home, school, or place of work. The latter practice yields much information not available to professionals who confine their activities to their offices, information from the client's environment which is often necessary for an adequate formulation of the presented problem and for adequate mobilization of resources to solve it.

An interview provides a more or less structured means of gathering information and can be general and wide-ranging or very detailed and specific. Interviews frequently bring up information that results in investigations by another professional person and another interview.

Medical Specialty Examinations

Man is a complex organism whose behavior has biological, developmental, sociocultural, and psychological aspects. Many mental health professionals believe that any diagnostic activity must include contributions from specialists in each of these areas. Man as an organism forms the special province of medicine and its various specialties. The functioning of certain parts of the body is related to behavior, and these physical aspects will often be examined in the mental health diagnostic process. This process will frequently include referral to a neurologist, a physician who is specially trained in the complex functioning of the nervous system, the sense organs, and the various glands that affect behavior.

Neurological Examinations

Organic diseases of the central nervous system may cause both behavioral and neurological symptoms. In addition to understanding the functions and dysfunctions of the mind, the psychiatrist has knowledge of the structure of the nervous system and the diseases that affect it. For this reason, most psychiatrists must have basic training in neurology. They may want to perform a neurological examination of their patient, or they may insist that such an examination be performed by a neurologist. Neurological examinations are quite standardized and routine medical procedures.

When a psychiatrist or neurologist conducts an examination his first task is to determine whether the condition he is investigating is due to organic or to psychological causes. If he determines that the cause of the condition is organic, the presumed cause and its location within the nervous system must be established.

An adequate personal history is probably the most important step in establishing a diagnosis and helping to differentiate neurological from psychological illness. The essential feature of such a history is a detailed time sequence of the development of the condition. The psychiatrist or neurologist investigates the condition with regard to its onset, duration, and frequency of occurrence. He may ask the patient a long and detailed series of questions about neurological symptoms to insure that nothing has been overlooked. Typical questions might be about whether the patient has experienced dizziness, headaches, episodes of fainting, fits or convulsions, shaking, trembling, unsteadiness or incoordination, weakness, stiffness, a paralysis, aches, pains, lack of sensation, numbness, double vision, spots before the eyes, temporary blindness, or blurred vision. Other questions which may seem unusual to a patient having his first neurological examination concern ringing in the ears, impairment of taste or smell, or hearing or seeing things that are out of the ordinary. Disturbances of swallowing or speech or an alteration of bowel or bladder control might also be important neurological symptoms. For women, details about pregnancy and menstruation might also be significant. Changes in sexual potency or recent variations in sexual activity might also be important features of the history. Alterations in sleep patterns, in addition to memory impairment, confusion, personality change, anxiety, or behavior that may be labeled "delinquent" might also prove to be symptoms of either neurological or psychological disturbance.

The neurologist also asks questions about traumatic events like surgery, head injuries, or other physical illnesses like diabetes or hypertension. He may ask about allergies, exposure to toxic substances, and gains or losses of weight. Additional questions concern the use of drugs or medication and past hospitalizations. The neurologist may inquire about more personal activities like occupation or drinking and smoking habits. He may ask a series of questions about venereal disease. Finally, he may inquire about other family members who have had diseases similar to the one the patient is presenting or about other congenital conditions. A general physical examination is always considered a routine part of the neurological examination. After the general physical examination comes the specific neurological examination, in which many seemingly unusual tests are conducted. In this part of the examination, the physician looks for alertness, degree of attention or distractibility, cooperativeness, and orientation to time, place, and person. He investigates the patient's memory with regard to both remote and recent events. He examines the patient's ability in attention and immediate recall, in performing calculations, and in dealing with abstract concepts. Since speech disturbances are also important, the neurologist may ask the patient to carry out certain tests which allow him to evaluate both spoken and written language. The physician also tries to find out if the patient can understand the examiner, asking him to repeat certain words or phrases. Can the patient pick out or point to an object that is named? Can he recognize familiar sounds? All of these are part of the neurologist's questioning repertoire.

The neurologist carries out specific examinations of the head and neck, checking the cranial nerves. He seeks answers to such questions as: Can the patient identify familiar odors? What is his visual acuity? Do the eyes move properly and do the pupils constrict with light and dark? Does he have sensation over the face and cornea? Does he have strength in his facial muscles? Can he hear adequately? Does he experience any nausea or dizziness as a result of the introduction of some ice water into the external ear canal? Will he gag when a tongue depressor is put into his throat? Can he raise his shoulders and lower them? Can the tongue be protruded normally and moved from side to side?

The next part of the neurological examination involves what is commonly called the motor examination. In this process the physician checks for posture, contractures and deformities of the extremities or trunk, muscle tenderness and strength, muscle tone, resistance to passive movement, and rigidity in the muscles, as well as voluntary muscle strength. He also looks for any involuntary movements. In a condition known as "Parkinsonism," for example, one of the characteristic features is a resting, rhythmic tremor affecting the extremities (particularly a circular motion of the thumb and fingers that resembles "pill-rolling").

Equilibrity, or the ability to keep one's balance, is examined next. The physician observes the patient walking normally, on his toes, and on his heels. He notes, further, the patient's ability to stand up with his eyes closed and his arms extended.

The sensory phase of the examination is often the most difficult and frustrating for both physician and patient. Both must be alert and cooperative. The physician usually sticks the patient with a pin to see if he can differentiate pain from touch sensations. He will also test the patient's vibratory sensation (by touching him with a tuning fork) and his position sense (by slowly moving the patient's fingers or toes). Last of all, the reflexes are tested, usually by tapping with a small, rubber-tipped hammer a tendon or bony prominence associated with a specific muscle. Superficial reflexes are tested by stroking the skin with a semi-sharp object.

A child's neurological examination is similar to that of an adult but has a different emphasis. The review of symptoms will prove less informative to the physician in the child's case, and the social history will concentrate more on environmental factors. The family history must be more thorough, and great importance is given to events before, during, and immediately following the child's birth. With infants, the essential objective of a neurological examination is the assessment of the maturity of the young patient in relation to that of his peers. The neurologist usually requires repeated observations before drawing any conclusions.

The EEG (electroencephalogram). Special laboratory tests are usually employed for the neurological examination. The diagnostic measure most commonly used by a neurologist is electroencephalography, which records the electrical activity of the brain. In preparation for taking the EEG, the patient is usually put in a very quiet room to rest. Superficial electrodes are attached to different parts of his scalp by means of a special paste. Some EEG administrations employ very fine needles which are inserted just under the skin of the patient's scalp. This procedure may cause a bit of discomfort but its advantage is that the results are clearer than those obtained with the paste method. The entire procedure takes about thirty minutes.

Different electrical activity of the brain is identifiable by various types of waves (some slower or faster, others of greater or lesser intensity). The interpretation of an EEG record is in large part impressionistic because the technician who reads the EEG records scans the entire record strip as a single picture rather than evaluating each individual wave.

There are no EEG patterns that are characteristic of only one specific disease (with the possible exception of certain forms of epilepsy). The response of cerebral electrical activity to injury of any type is relatively limited; the cause of the injury will have little bearing on the test results. The EEG helps the physician to evaluate brain tumors, lesions of the blood vessels of the brain, inflammatory diseases of the brain (like abscesses or infections), trauma to the brain, degenerative diseases involving losses of brain tissue, and epilepsy. But since the EEG can sometimes miss certain kinds of brain disorders, different kinds of additional techniques may have to be used to detect those abnormalities.

It should be pointed out that except in certain cases of epilepsy, the EEG is usually not a definitive test but only one of many laboratory tools. The neurologist uses its findings in association with all other factors in the clinical evaluation of the patient.

Examination of spinal fluid. Another very important test for neurological evaluation (and we must keep in mind that neurological disorders can cause changes in behavior patterns) is examination of the spinal fluid. The spinal tap is performed under sterile conditions by inserting a needle into the spinal canal below the spinal cord which ends near the so-called small of the back. A local anesthetic is used so that the patient does not have discomfort during the procedure. For the spinal tap the patient is sometimes asked to lie on his side, curled up with his knees touching his chest. Other physicians prefer to do the examination with the patient sitting on the table.

The physician measures the spinal fluid pressure and examines the color and clarity of the fluid. The spinal fluid is routinely examined at the laboratory for both red and white cells, serology (tests for venereal disease), protein, and sugar. The results of these laboratory tests are important because they can indicate to the neurologist the presence of certain diseases.

Skull X rays.   X rays (roentgenograms) of the skull are also very helpful to the neurologist in making a diagnosis of central nervous system disease. Routine X rays of the skull include front, back, and side views and special views of the head with the chin flexed on the chest. Skull X rays are most helpful in identifying conditions like calcifications or erosions of the skull and areas of bony protrusions.

Brain scans.   Neurologists also use another radiographic technique commonly known as the brain scan. This technique consists in injecting radioisotopic material into a vein two to four hours before a scanning device takes pictures of the brain. During the process the patient usually rests comfortably on the table and photographic equipment passes back and forth over the skull, usually for a period of about an hour. Abnormal tissue within the head (in contrast to normal brain tissue) tends to retain the radioisotopic compounds, and this enables the radiologist to arrive at an accurate diagnosis. The brain scan is extremely useful in helping to localize lesions in the brain such as tumors, abscesses, and blood clots.

Echoencephalography.   Another diagnostic procedure which is becoming popular is echoencephalography. In this technique, recorded echoes of very-high-frequency sound (ultrasound) are used to measure the location of structures within the brain. This test is administered in a manner similar to the brain scan, but without the use of the radioisotopic injection. The procedure is painless and can be used as a screening procedure in cases of suspected mass lesions inside the skull.

Pneumoencephalography.   Pneumoencephalography makes it possible for the neurologist to visualize areas normally containing spinal fluid. The same technique is used as in drawing spinal fluid except that air is introduced into the spinal canal. X rays are then taken and the air is seen in contrast with the brain and bone tissue, enabling the physician to arrive at an accurate diagnosis.

Myelography.   Myelography is a procedure similar to pneumoencephalography in that a radio-opaque dye is injected into the spinal canal by means of a puncture in the lower part of the back. Since the radio-opaque solution is heavier than the spinal fluid, it can be maneuvered throughout the spinal canal by having the patient tilted on the x-ray table. Lesions of the spinal canal can then be precisely located by means of x-ray and fluoroscope records.

Angiograms. The last of the specific tests is cerebral angiography. In this procedure the neurologist introduces a radio-opaque solution into the arteries supplying the brain so that these may then be visualized in cerebral x-ray studies.

Biopsies. In very rare circumstances a biopsy (the removal of small bits of tissue for analysis) may be made of nervous system tissue. This procedure is carried out primarily when possible lesions are easily accessible, such as when they are located in the spinal canal.

There are, of course, specific situations that require the employment of the different techniques described above. The neurologist will determine which of these tests to use in each particular case in order to reach an accurate diagnosis.

Psychological Tests

The diagnostic procedure very often involves the use of a wide variety of psychological tests, which are standardized tasks constructed and administered in such a way that the taker's performance can be compared with the performance of other persons or groups doing the same task. The purpose of these tests is to allow the psychologist to make a controlled and standardized observation of some aspect of the test taker's mental functioning. The psychologist may wish to observe language ability, reading comprehension, vocational interests, level of social sensitivity, or any number of other mental or intellectual functions. Of course no one can directly observe an "attitude" or an "aptitude" since these terms are really concepts rather than concrete things or events. The existence of an attitude, for example, is inferred by the observer on the basis of some observable behavior, in this case the test taker's performance on the various test items. Since there is always a level of uncertainty in making inferences about anything, psychological tests are valuable to mental health professionals because they attempt to reduce this uncertainty to a minimum by holding the behavioral observations as constant as possible from test taker to test taker. This feature of psychological tests gives the psychologist two important advantages. First, it allows him to learn from experience by enabling him to compare the accuracy of inferences he has made in the past with the actual outcomes of those cases. Second, given a question answerable by test results, he can save both the client and himself time by making controlled behavior observations in the least possible time. The usefulness of the test results is based on the assumption that performance on the test bears some relationship to behavior in nontest situations.

The psychologist is trained to administer many different types of psychological tests, and to analyze the results. One of the most important things for the psychologist to know is which tests to use in each situation. Psychological tests are sometimes administered in a *battery* (a group of psychological tests given to an individual over a relatively short period of time) in order to answer a specific question or series of questions. Some of the general types of psychological tests follow.

Personality tests. Personality can be defined as the sum of the patterns and qualities of the behavior of a particular person. Personality tests enable the psychologist to conceptualize the personality or various aspects of it. Some of these aspects are attitudes toward authority figures, the quality of various interpersonal relationships, and likely reactions to certain kinds of stresses.

The formats of the various personality tests are quite diverse and can include tasks like drawing figures, responding to "inkblots," or answering a long series of true-false questions. Some tests have rather elaborate and complex scoring schemes; others are interpreted quite impressionistically. In any event, personality tests are usually designed to allow the psychologist to make inferences both about *what* the test taker does (on the task items), and about *how* he does it. In this respect, just about any standardized set of task items can be used as a personality test by a skilled psychologist.

Intelligence tests. Intelligence can be broadly defined as the ability to acquire and retain knowledge and to respond quickly and successfully to new situations. In this respect there are really many different kinds of intelligence: the ability to use words, the ability to use numbers, the ability to coordinate the hands and eyes, and so forth. As a general rule, intelligence tests measure one or more of these specific abilities and the results of the test for a given person are expressed as a comparison between that individual's performance and the performance of a large number of people (of similar chronological age or educational level) on the same test.

Intelligence tests are usually comprised of graded items—that is, a series of task items of progressively increasing difficulty. As the test taker proceeds through the test, the items become harder and harder until a point is reached where he is unable to answer a large proportion of the items correctly. This point, which marks the test taker's *mental age,* is compared with the test taker's chronological age, or his actual age in years and months. If his performance has been average for his age group, his mental age divided by his chronological age will be 1.0—that is, they will be the same. The number representing the comparison between mental age and chronological age is called the *intelligence quotient,* or I.Q. It is computed as follows:

$$\text{I.Q.} = \frac{\text{mental age}}{\text{chronological age}} \times 100.$$

(The comparison of the two ages is multiplied by 100 to avoid dealing with decimals.) If a person has a mental age greater than his chronological age, his intelligence quotient would be greater than 100, or above average. If his mental age is less than his chronological age, his I.Q. would be less than 100. (On most I.Q. tests "average" is expressed as a range of scores, for example, the range between scores of 90 and 110.)

There are many kinds of intelligence tests. Some tap a wide variety of intellectual skills whereas others test only one specific ability, like verbal skill. These tests can be administered to individuals or to groups of people together, as in schools or in military service.

Standardized intelligence tests have been widely criticized on the grounds that they measure intellectual achievement rather than intellectual ability. The most frequent criticism states that since some of these abilities are more common in certain socioeconomic groups than in others, the tests are not fair to the groups in which these skills are less common. This argument has much to recommend it and work is proceeding on the development of tests that measure ability regardless of the language or cultural background of the test taker. It will probably be some time before such culture-free intelligence tests can be developed and put into common use.

Social competence tests. Tests of social maturity are used mainly with young children and occasionally with older persons who are mentally retarded. They are designed to compare the activity of an individual with the similar performance of a large number of people in his same age group. Social maturity is measured by surveying the social skills the individual has acquired at a given age. Examples of social skills are feeding oneself, dressing oneself, and so forth. An interesting aspect of some tests of social maturity is that the mother or someone else who is in a position to observe the child closely serves as a reporter and completes the test items.

Educational achievement tests. Tests of educational achievement are most commonly used within school systems. Usually administered to all students about every two years, these tests are conducted in a group setting, often the homeroom class. The results are presented as the grade level at which the student is performing across a number of academic subjects, and are then entered in the student's record as a profile of his academic progress.

Vocational and interest tests. Several kinds of vocational and interest tests are used by counseling psychologists to obtain information about the abilities, attributes, and values of the client. The results enable the counselor to guide the client toward a more satisfying vocation or to a style of living which better suits his personality. Only two types of vocational tests will be discussed here.

First, there are tests of specific abilities that are related and necessary to success in a particular occupation. A good example of this is a test of manual dexterity. In such a test the test taker's ability to manipulate objects and to solve mechanical problems are closely observed and matched against the performance of an occupational reference group. In order to be a successful mechanic, watchmaker, or dentist, a high level of manual dexterity is required. A clerk, librarian, or attorney would not need such a high level in order to pursue his profession, but he would require a high level of reading comprehension. The purpose of these tests, then, is to match the individual with the occupation in terms of basic skill requirements.

Sociocultural Diagnosis and Social Work

Diagnosing the sociocultural aspects of the client's behavior is within the area of competence of the social worker. Adequate understanding of the client as a social and cultural being requires that an accurate word picture of him be painted against an equally detailed background of his complex life situation. The result of this process is a survey of the multiple relationships that exist between the client and his environment. These include family, school, work, church, civic, and myriad other relationships in which the client may be involved. Some may be problematic and, consequently, the subjects of therapeutic effort; others may emerge as strengths to be utilized in the treatment process. The relationships between the client and his environment may be constructed either currently and/or historically.

The case history. To get an understanding of a mental problem being presented to him, the professional (frequently a social worker) constructs a systematic account of the development of the problem over some period of time with the help of the client. This systematic reconstruction of past events is called a *history.*

Sometimes it seems to the client that the historical facts the professional is interested in are not directly related to the present and pressing problem he is experiencing. Many behavior problems, however, are believed to originate in early childhood or in the client's social circumstances long before the present difficulty was recognized as such by the client. Also, because the social worker is looking for strengths as well as weaknesses in the client's situation, the construction of the history deals with more than currently problematic issues.

Sources of current situational information. A comprehensive picture of the client's present situation requires timely and accurate information from many sources. First, of course, is the client himself. The mental health professional interviews him to obtain a picture of his present circumstances, especially an indication of how the client himself views them. In addition to the factual information, the interviewer pays particular attention to what the client does and does not relate about his current situation, to what he thinks is important, and so forth.

Diagnostic interviews may include people other than the client. Since the purpose of a social case history is to yield a picture of the client's life circumstances, interviews may be scheduled with his spouse, parents, or other family members—with the client's permission, of course.

Case records research. Valuable diagnostic information relating to the client, such as hospital or school records, may already have been collected by another diagnostic or treatment agency. Mental health professionals frequently ask the client's permission (in writing) to obtain such information. This permission is usually called an *information release,* and the form that the client is asked to sign stipulates the source from which the information is to be requested, as well as certifies that the information, once obtained, will be used for professional purposes only and that it will be treated as confidential. Reviewing previous records for diagnostic purposes can be seen as a kind of remote interview.

Certain current and very specific information about the presented problem or about some aspect of it may be deemed necessary to the diagnostic process. This information usually serves as a baseline against which later treatment efforts will be compared, and it often takes the form of behavior records kept by the client and submitted to the mental health professional at specified intervals. These records may include behaviors like the time of retiring or awaking, the time spent studying, or the number of task units accomplished in some unit of time. The responsibility of the client for keeping such records can also be viewed as a kind of remote-controlled extension of the diagnostic interview.

The Team Approach to Diagnosis

Defining a mental problem in such a way that something can be done about it is a complicated task, because all human behavior, problematic and otherwise, is influenced by many causes. One way of classifying the causes of human behavior is to divide them into biological, psychological-developmental, and sociocultural categories. This is an especially convenient classification of the causes of human behavior for our purposes here, because it parallels the particular areas of competence of the three mental health professions—psychiatry, psychology, and social work. The very natural way that the professional activities of these groups complement one another in the defining of mental disorders accounts for the fact that we so frequently find a psychiatrist, a psychologist, and a social worker functioning as a diagnostic team.

CHAPTER 4

Treatment: Solving Mental Problems

Psychological Treatment: Psychotherapy

The term *psychotherapy* is difficult to define in a simple yet accurate way. Two good definitions borrowed from highly respected professional references are:

Broadly considered, psychotherapy includes all methods for modifying disturbed behavior by psychological means.[1]

and

[Psychotherapy] is a form of treatment for problems of an emotional nature in which a trained person deliberately establishes a professional relationship with a patient with the object of removing, modifying, or retarding existing symptoms, or mediating disturbed patterns of behavior, and of promoting positive personality growth and development.[2]

The awesome complexity of the human mind and our vast ignorance about how it functions have provided the necessary conditions for the development of many different kinds of psychotherapy. In 1959 Robert A. Harper published a book describing thirty-six different systems of psychotherapy.[3] The last decade has witnessed the development of

1. H. A. Storrow, *Outline of Clinical Psychiatry* (New York: Appleton-Century-Crofts, 1969), p. 347.
2. L. R. Worlberg, *The Technique of Psychotherapy* (New York: Grune & Stratton, 1954). Quoted in L. E. Hinsie and R. J. Campbell, eds., *Psychiatric Dictionary,* 3rd ed. (New York: Oxford University Press, 1960), p. 630.
3. R. A. Harper, *Psychoanalysis and Psychotherapy—36 Systems* (Englewood Cliffs, N.J.: Prentice-Hall, 1959).

many additional types, schools, or systems of psychotherapy, and the list is still growing. Each system of psychotherapy is based on a particular theory of human behavior. These theories are sets of more or less organized ideas about the causes of both normal and abnormal behavior. As a result, each system of psychotherapy defines and attempts to modify various aspects of human behavior according to its underlying theory. Each system defines its treatment goals, clients, practitioners, techniques, and results in its own particular way. And, of course, each system of psychotherapy has its supporters in both the professional and client communities.

For all their diversity, the various systems of psychotherapy do seem to have some important things in common. As Singer has pointed out, "there is a single proposition which underlies all forms of psychotherapy: the proposition that *man is capable of change and capable of bringing this change about himself,* provided he is aided in his search of such change."[4] Each system of psychotherapy seems to produce positive results for some of the people who use it. And most important, no single system of psychotherapy works for all people or all problems. In fact, all the psychotherapy systems combined can adequately describe only a fraction of the problematic behavior that can be directly observed.

In a book of this length it would be impossible to describe even a few systems of psychotherapy in detail.[5] For the purposes of this discussion, however, the various systems of psychotherapy can be divided into two general classes: insight-centered psychotherapies and behavior-centered psychotherapies.

Insight-centered Psychotherapies

Insight-centered psychotherapies have as their primary goal the increasing of the patient's understanding of (or insight into) his own behavior. Several systems within this group of psychotherapies are

4. E. Singer, *Key Concepts in Psychotherapy* (New York: Random House, 1965), p. 16.
5. Readers who are interested in studying one or more of these systems should consult the references cited in the notes for this chapter.

based on what are called *dynamic* theories of behavior, which deal with the ways that the personality develops over time. The dynamic behavior theories generally view both normal and abnormal behavior as a *symptom* of some deeper, unobservable cause.

The psychotherapies founded upon dynamic behavior theories concentrate on discovering the underlying causes of behavior and on increasing the patient's insights about these causes. Many such theories assert that events occurring in early childhood (*causes*) exert a powerful influence upon later adult behavior (*symptoms*). The emphasis on the distinction between symptoms and underlying causes has suggested to some people that these systems of psychotherapy are based upon a *medical model* (or design) of treatment. The influence of medical practice on these systems of psychotherapy is further suggested by the use of the term *therapy* itself, by the description of abnormal behavior as psycho*pathology*, and by identifying the person who is receiving the treatment as a *patient*.

Several kinds of insight-centered psychotherapy are widely accepted practices in the United States today. Some of these are: classical or Freudian psychoanalysis, analytic psychology, dynamic-cultural psychoanalytic methods, psychoanalytically oriented psychotherapy, analytic group therapy, existential analysis, and client-centered therapy. Probably the most popular example of an insight-centered system of psychotherapy is classical or Freudian psychoanalysis.

Psychoanalysis. It is commonly said that psychoanalysis is the application of the therapist's "microscope" to events in the patient's life, particularly those which took place during early childhood. Therefore, psychoanalysis is an investigative procedure. It makes a thorough examination of the individual during sessions that take place up to four or five times a week for a year or more.

Psychoanalysis is a psychological method of treatment founded on the theories of Sigmund Freud. It is expensive and time-consuming, is applicable only to a number of carefully selected patients, and, like other methods, it has its limitations. There are several systems of psychotherapy that are modifications of psychoanalysis. These are based on different theoretical approaches to the problems presented by patients.

A psychoanalyst does not necessarily need to be a psychiatrist, that is, a physician, as required by the American Psychoanalytic Association. As a matter of fact, Freud was in favor of training nonmedical psychoanalysts; his daughter, Anna, considered one of the world's most prominent psychoanalysts, is not a physician. Most psychoanalysts in the United States, however, are psychiatrists. Whatever the professional background of the psychoanalyst, it is required that he have special advanced training in the practice of psychoanalysis and must, in addition, have spent several years in his own personal psychoanalysis.

Behavior-centered Psychotherapies

Behavior-centered psychotherapies seek to bring about the direct modification of some specific aspect of the client's behavior. Many systems within this group of psychotherapies are based upon what are commonly called *learning theories,* which generally view both normal and abnormal behavior as resulting from the influence of contingencies in the client's immediate environment. Learning theories (and the psychotherapeutic systems on which they are based) hold that specific behavior patterns can be modified by identifying and altering the environmental factors associated with them.

Because they concentrate on directly observable behavior and events, these systems of psychotherapy are sometimes referred to as *behavior modification* or *contingency management* systems. They are sometimes classified as *social model* systems because they emphasize the client's immediate environment without regard to underlying causes of behavior.

Although the various behavior modification techniques are sometimes called therapies, the person who receives the treatment is usually called a client. The person who administers the treatment is usually referred to as a teacher or trainer. The particular behavior at which the treatment is directed is called a *target* behavior, instead of psychopathology.

Some of the systems of psychotherapy that might be classified as behavior-centered are: assertion-structured psychotherapy, fixed-role therapy, hypnotherapy, implosive therapy, psychodrama, reciprocal-inhibition therapy, rational-emotive therapy, and reinforcement therapy. The last, particularly, is typical of the behavior-centered group of psychotherapies.

Reinforcement therapy. One of the most influential of the behavior-centered psychotherapies is called *operant conditioning*. The theory behind this system was developed by Professor B. F. Skinner of Harvard University. According to this theory, a subject "operates" upon his environment by behaving in a certain way. The way the environment responds to (or reinforces) this behavior has an important influence upon the future behavior of the subject.

The psychotherapy system based on this theory involves the identification of specific problematic behaviors and the specific environmental responses (reinforcements) related to them. With this information the trainer devises a plan to systematically change these reinforcements in such a way that the target behavior is modified or changed. Clients of this form of psychotherapy are encouraged to take an active part in the treatment process by keeping records of their progress, usually in the form of charts and graphs.

Like all other psychotherapies, reinforcement therapy works better for some people and some problems than it does for others. Because this form of psychotherapy is administered in a relatively short series of sessions, it is a correspondingly inexpensive method of treatment.

Some Methods of Delivering Psychotherapeutic Treatment

Certain forms of psychotherapy are best described in terms of the time it takes to accomplish them and the setting in which they are used. For example, brief psychotherapy is a method of administering psychotherapeutic treatment in a very short period of time. Because it represents a method of delivering treatment rather than a particular system of treatment, it could be based on either an insight-oriented or a behavior-oriented system of psychotherapy. The distinguishing feature of this method is that its course is abbreviated.

Group psychotherapy and family therapy are methods of administering psychotherapy to more than one person at a time. Their distinguishing feature is the setting (a group of people) in which the treatment occurs.

Brief psychotherapy. Many people believe that psychotherapy always has to be a long and expensive process. Although this may be true for some individuals suffering from certain mental disorders, it is definitely not true for all persons experiencing mental or emotional difficulties.

Brief psychotherapy is a much foreshortened application of traditional psychotherapy selected because of the life situation of the patient or because of the setting in which the treatment is offered. Emergency psychotherapy is brief psychotherapy applied in special situations of crisis and exigency.[6] In many cases, ten to twelve sessions are adequate for the therapist to deal effectively with the current stressful life situations of the patient. It should be emphasized that brief psychotherapy is not the treatment of choice for best handling all cases of mental disorder and that a careful assessment of the individual's problem by a competent therapist is of vital importance in deciding whether a person will profit from this method.

The establishment of mental health centers, walk-in emergency clinics, student health services, and other types of easily accessible community facilities has helped the development of brief psychotherapy as a partial solution to the huge problem of delivering mental health services. Brief psychotherapy is gaining greater public acceptance because it usually yields positive results, it represents a significant saving of time and money, and it accommodates the right of all people to receive timely mental health service when they need it. One of the most important aspects of the widespread application of brief psychotherapy is that it can help many people avoid the necessity of a future long-term course of psychotherapy or, in some cases, residential treatment in a mental hospital.

Group psychotherapy. In group psychotherapy the principles of treatment are applied to several persons meeting at the same time. The individual patient (or client) and other members of the group enter into an agreement with the therapist to meet with him at certain times, in a given place and for a specified number of sessions. The therapist carefully screens and selects group members who, in his opinion, are likely to profit from the collective psychotherapy experience. Once the group is organized, the members and the therapist can set up certain rules in addition to those stipulated by the therapist in the beginning.

Sometimes there are two or more therapists, either of the same or opposite sex. Both therapists could be active participants in the group's

6. L. Bellak and L. Small, *Emergency Psychotherapy and Brief Psychotherapy* (New York: Grune & Stratton, 1965), pp. 6–10.

discussions, or one of them might function as an observer, taking notes and generally acting as the recording secretary of the sessions.

The system of psychotherapy employed in the group setting depends on the therapist's training, skills, and preferred system of treatment. The system or model of group therapy to be used is usually explained to the group members, whose participation and cooperation are essential for success.

A common goal of group psychotherapy is the improvement of communication within the group in order to reduce the isolation of the individual members while providing them with some useful insights into their individual interpersonal conflicts and difficulties. By sharing personal experiences with other members of the group they facilitate interaction among one another for the purpose of ultimately improving their relationships with other persons outside of the group.

Group psychotherapy should be distinguished from other group techniques currently used for educational or training purposes in industry, schools, and other organizations. Examples of such techniques are: (1) sensitivity, personal encounter, or "t" groups (the *t* standing for training), (2) task-oriented groups, and (3) intervention laboratories. Although some authors claim that there is not a clear-cut distinction between sensitivity training and psychotherapy, others[7] have pointed to "typical differences" regarding the selection of participants, group goals and leadership, duration of the group's activities, relationship between the group members, and the content of the discussions that take place within the groups.

Throughout the last decade group activities have proliferated in all parts of the United States. Unfortunately, not a few unskilled charlatans have been making a great business using so-called group techniques. This situation can cause a great deal of harm to legions of uninformed people who are seeking to relieve their emotional problems through a legitimate group psychotherapy experience. The credentials of a potential group leader should be investigated before making a contract to participate in his group.

Family therapy.　　The need to involve the entire family as a unit in

7. L. A. Gottschalk and E. M. Pattison, "Psychiatric Perspectives on T-Groups and the Laboratory Movement: An Overview," *American Journal of Psychiatry* 126, no. 6 (December 1969): 823–39.

the psychotherapeutic process was realized many years ago as a result of observations made in child guidance clinics. It was recognized that, in addition to the mother, other members of a young patient's family could contribute to the understanding and solution of the problem the patient was presenting. "Interest was broadened to diagnosing and treating the family as a unit, since the difficulties of the referred child were seen as one sign of a general disturbance."[8] Nowadays, the identified patient could be any member of the family and not necessarily the child whose difficulties initiated the family therapeutic process.

A good, concise description of family therapy is found in the following paragraph from *The Field of Family Therapy,* a report produced by the Group for the Advancement of Psychiatry (GAP):

Family therapy today is not a treatment method in the usual sense; there is no generally-agreed-upon set of procedures followed by practitioners who consider themselves family therapists. What these practitioners hold in common is the premise that psychopathology in an individual may be an expression of family pathology and the conviction that seeing a family together may offer advantages over seeing its members individually. From these basic views various kinds of therapeutic intervention can emerge, and all of them must be considered family therapy. Some family therapists will interview only the whole family; others will see pairs of individuals as well as the whole group; still others typically see only an individual but with the goal of changing family context so that he can change."[9]

Describing the professional background of people carrying out family therapy, the GAP report states further that in their questionnaire sample "social workers make up the largest single group, about 40 percent, and psychiatrists and psychologists together account for another 40 percent. Among the remaining are marriage counselors, clergymen, nonpsychiatric physicians, child psychiatrists, nurses, sociologists, and others from scattered disciplines."[10]

Initial Contact and Interview with a Psychotherapist

A person may seek help from a psychotherapist on his own initiative, or as a referral from a professional person, or on the recommendation

8. Committee on the Family, Group for the Advancement of Psychiatry, *The Field of Family Therapy,* no. 79 (March 1970): 572.
9. Ibid.
10. Ibid.

of a friend, relative, clergyman, or colleague. There are people who do not come to the psychotherapist voluntarily but, rather, come under some legal or other coercion. A judge, for example, might propose "the alternative of psychotherapy" to a defendant as a condition of probation. The same alternative might be proposed by a board of parole to a convict seeking release from prison. Various forms of psychotherapy (brief, group, etc.) are used in correctional systems when patients (offenders) become engaged in treatment either because they are legally committed to do so, because they were advised to do so by someone, or simply because they are voluntarily seeking help for themselves.

The initial contact with the therapist may take place as a face-to-face meeting, or via a written letter or telephone call. The initial interview takes place during the first scheduled appointment. By the end of the interview the therapist usually has an idea about the most suitable type of treatment the prospective patient is likely to require, depending upon his particular needs, age, intelligence, environment, and economic situation. An important factor, of course, is the therapist's individual training and his preferred method of treatment. If the therapist decides that specific diagnostic work is needed at this point, he may refer the patient to an appropriate professional person for this purpose before making any further decision about the course of therapy.

The Psychotherapeutic Contract

Further interviews and decisions about the method of treatment require a verbal agreement between the patient (or client) and the therapist. (A written agreement is seldom used.) The agreement between the therapist and the patient concerning the ground rules of the therapy is known as the therapeutic contract or, simply, the contract.

The contract outlines in detail the responsibilities of both patient and therapist in such a way that each knows what he has a right to expect of the other during the course of the therapy. The therapist specifies the times he will reserve for the patient (the hour and the day of the week on which the sessions will be held). He also indicates the length of the interviews (thirty minutes, fifty minutes, etc.), the frequency of appointments (once a week, once every other week, etc.), where the appointments will take place, the duration of treatment, fees, and method of payment. In addition, the therapist stipulates some minimal rules for the sessions. These rules might include prohibitions against physical assaults and the destruction of property within the therapist's office. Contractual items may also be specified by the patient. Examples of these items might be a commitment to a certain number of sessions, a commitment to reevaluate the progress of the psychotherapy at certain time intervals, agreement on the kind and amount of behavior change to be used in the evaluation of the therapy, and agreement about what will be done if the therapy is successful or not successful according to the predetermined criteria (such options could include termination of the therapy, continuation of the therapy, or referral to another practitioner).

After the patient and the therapist have negotiated a therapeutic contract acceptable to both of them, they may consider it to be binding. Patients (or clients) should beware of therapeutic contracts which contain rules stipulated only by the therapist, or those which do not contain specific provisions for periodic reevaluation of the progress of the therapy.

Psychotherapy and Other Forms of Treatment

Psychotherapy can be, and often is, combined with other forms of treatment in an individual treatment plan. The prescription of medication or a regimen of electroconvulsive therapy (ECT) are methods that are often combined with psychotherapy. Although any qualified mental health professional might be a psychotherapist, only a licensed physician can prescribe medication and other somatic (physical) treatment for patients.

Drug Treatment: Chemotherapy

Frequently used in psychiatric treatment, drugs can exert very potent actions affecting both feelings and behavior. The many different kinds of drugs working in various areas of the brain may be classified as (1) major tranquilizers, (2) minor tranquilizers, (3) major stimulants, and (4) minor stimulants.

Major Tranquilizers: Antipsychotic Drugs

The major tranquilizers produce a calming effect with a minimal impairment of the patient's intellectual functions. They are prescribed by physicians for patients who exhibit signs of serious anxiety, overactivity, agitation, thinking disturbances, and certain patterns of withdrawn or underactive behavior. In some patients these drugs may produce minor to severe side effects such as motor restlessness, muscle spasms (lasting from several seconds to several minutes), tremors, unusual body postures, or unusual facial expressions. If side effects occur, the physician may prescribe other medications to correct them.

Minor Tranquilizers: Antianxiety Drugs

The minor tranquilizers produce a calming effect with less likelihood of creating a state of confusion than is the case with other nonselective central nervous system depressants such as barbiturates. The relatively wide range between the therapeutic and lethal doses of these drugs makes them safer to use with suicide-risk patients than the nonselective depressants. Minor tranquilizers are prescribed by physicians for patients exhibiting mild or moderate signs of anxiety and agitation. They are relatively ineffective with more severe disturbances.

Another group of minor tranquilizers are the nonselective central nervous system depressants, which include barbiturates and nonbarbiturate sedatives. These drugs are likely to produce confusion in doses adequate to calm anxious patients, and therefore some physicians find them less useful than other minor tranquilizers. The barbiturates and other nonbarbiturate sedatives all are capable of producing addiction. Since they are the drugs most commonly used in suicide attempts physicians prescribe them with caution and in small quantities.

Major Stimulants: Mood Elevators

The major stimulants, sometimes called mood elevators, are prescribed for patients who exhibit a depressed mood and its associated symptoms, especially lethargy and decreased activity. Because these drugs have a delay in producing their therapeutic effect, they are used with caution for patients who appear to be serious suicide risks.

Minor Stimulants: Antidepressants

The minor stimulants have more of a direct stimulative than anti-depressant effect. Some of them have been found useful in the treatment of overactive children. Physicians do not prescribe this medication for severely depressed patients because the drugs sometimes have a tendency to produce or increase agitation and overactivity. Furthermore, chronic overdose of these drugs may cause severe emotional disturbances requiring hospitalization.

Important Note About Drugs and Medications

All drugs and medications should be used only under the proper guidance and direction of a physician. Aside from the legal prohibitions against unauthorized drug use, there are two very compelling reasons for adhering to this principle religiously:

1. There is more to obtaining the desired effect from a drug than simply taking a pill. The reliably therapeutic effect of any medication can be achieved only when the chemical characteristics of the drug, the intricacies of the patient's physical condition, and the specific object of the therapy are known and considered wisely.
2. All drugs have the potential for producing severe side effects or unintended results. These effects can be precipitated by the patient's physical condition, by combination with other medications or foods, or by taking them in excessive dosages or over too long a period of time.

Somatic Therapies

Electroconvulsive Therapy (ECT)

Artificial convulsions are sometimes used as a treatment for certain kinds of mental disorders. In the past drugs were injected to induce these seizures. Now, however, the electric-current method has replaced the earlier techniques because the convulsions are more predictable and controllable, because the unconsciousness comes at once rather than after a delay, and because the method is safer than the use of injected drugs.

A grand mal convulsion (similar to an epileptic seizure) is induced by sending an electric current through the brain. The physician usually attempts to employ the smallest voltage for the shortest time period found adequate to produce a convulsion. The convulsion can be softened and the patient's fears reduced if the patient is sedated and if his muscular contractions are then diminished with an intravenous injection of a muscle relaxant. This adjustment can often be accomplished to the extent that the convulsions can be recognized only by looking carefully for minor contractions occurring in the small muscles of the hands and feet.

In addition to a convulsion, ECT brings about a period of unconsciousness which alone is not sufficient for producing the therapeutic effect. The convulsion is also necessary, but the precise mechanism for the therapeutic effect of ECT is not known.

Physicians recommend the use of ECT for patients exhibiting severe depression that has not responded to drugs. Certain other serious emotional disorders—for example, those of patients exhibiting an extremely agitated, overactive state which could be life threatening—are treated with ECT.

The side effect of ECT is impairment of memory, which can last for a few weeks or a few months. Permanent memory impairments resulting from ECT have not been demonstrated. The physician requires the patient to have a thorough physical examination before administering this therapy.

Insulin Coma Treatment

Insulin coma treatment was once a very popular method for treating the condition known as schizophrenia. Its effectiveness, however, has never been established, and those patients said to be most suitable for treatment by this method are also those most likely to improve with no treatment at all. Although insulin coma treatment is still popular in some European countries, its use has been almost entirely discontinued in the United States.

Psychosurgery: Lobotomy

Lobotomy is a surgical procedure that involves the interruption of the connection between certain brain structures related to emotional responses in the prefrontal area of the brain. The surgery is done in the operating room and it requires that the patient be anesthetized. The purpose of the psychosurgery is to reduce the intensity of the problematic emotional responses. It does not have a major influence on thinking. Although lobotomized patients often become less violent and easier to manage as a result of the procedure, a common side effect is a reduced ability to behave in other socially appropriate ways. Psychosurgery is a method for controlling rather than correcting behavior and the procedure is not reversible. Although rarely used today, it is occasionally advocated by some physicians for patients who are especially distressed and violent and who have failed to respond to all other treatment methods.

CHAPTER 5

Residential or Inpatient Treatment Facilities

Residential facilities are those in which the patient or client lives while he is receiving mental health services. Many general hospitals are able to provide residential or inpatient treatment in their psychiatric services, but mental hospitals are the most common example of this type of facility. Although there are several different kinds of mental hospitals, there exists one important variant: how much freedom and autonomy the resident has while he is receiving treatment. The point of comparison is the amount of freedom a given individual would have in his normal home or community life. Of course, this varies widely from individual to individual, depending on whether, for example, the patient is a child, the ward of a court, a soldier, or a civilian adult. Therefore, the treatment needs of the individual, his legal status when he accepts treatment, and the policies of the institution in which he seeks treatment are all important factors that will influence the patient's freedom of movement. These factors all relate to the patient's prerogatives to seek treatment, to initiate treatment, to engage in treatment, and finally, to terminate it.

Classification of Mental Hospitals

Probably the simplest way to classify mental hospitals is by their sponsorship. For our purposes here it will be sufficient to discuss three kinds of mental hospitals: (1) private mental hospitals, (2) public mental hospitals, and (3) teaching and research mental hospitals. There are variations, of course, but all mental hospitals should be accredited by the Joint Commission on Hospital Accreditation in the same way that general medical and surgical hospitals are accredited.

Private Mental Hospitals

Private mental hospitals operate in a manner similar to private general medical and surgical hospitals. Patients are accepted for treatment only if they are referred by a physician who has a contractual relationship with the hospital, if they are referrals from some locality or from some group such as a religious organization or labor union, or if they are subscribers of prepaying medical care and have been referred by a group-practice hospital. In all cases, however, the hospital charges for its services and a physician is ultimately responsible for entering the patient into the hospital.

Inpatient treatment in progressive private mental hospitals is expensive, sometimes costing $150 per day or more. The patient, his insurance company, or some group of which he is a member must bear this cost directly. (Although some private mental hospitals receive outside support to subsidize these expenses, we are discussing a purely private hospital here.) As a result, inpatient treatment in a private mental hospital tends to be relatively brief and intense. When long-term hospitalization is advised in a private mental hospital, the cost is prohibitive for most people. The trend today, however, is toward briefer periods of hospitalization in all types of mental hospitals.

The basic rates for treatment in a private mental hospital often include only the cost of residential treatment. Other items like medication and psychotherapy are frequently billed as separate items. These factors should be considered and discussed in the initial contract between the patient-to-be and the private hospital, a contract similar to that between patient and therapist.

Public Mental Hospitals

Various units of government operate and/or subsidize the operation of mental hospitals. Because these institutions are really subunits of the government, their staffs are usually made up of civil servants. Most public mental hospitals accept referrals from the particular geographic area they serve. Sometimes two or more cities or counties may jointly sponsor such a public mental hospital. In addition, an individual may be eligible to receive services in a U.S. Veterans Administration Hospital, but this requires a previous connection with the military service or certain branches of the government.

Treatment in public mental hospitals is also expensive, but all or most of the cost is subsidized by the unit of government that sponsors the hospital. Most public hospitals use a sliding-fee schedule in billing patients for diagnostic and treatment services. Under this system, the fee depends upon the patient's ability to pay. Patients with higher incomes pay relatively more, and those with lower incomes pay relatively less, or nothing at all. In any event, the cost to the patient for diagnostic and treatment services in a public mental hospital is decidedly less than in a comparable private institution.

Because of the cost differential between private and public mental hospitals, the public hospitals for years tended to be the repository of patients in need of long-term treatment, but this situation has been changing in recent years, owing largely to the introduction of community mental health centers. It sometimes happens, though, that a patient in need of long-term treatment will first receive inpatient treatment in a private mental hospital. Then, if the length of the treatment exceeds the limits of the patient's resources (insurance coverage, private funds, etc.) he may be transferred to a public facility for the remainder of his inpatient hospitalization.

Teaching and Research Mental Hospitals

Some mental hospitals train mental health professionals as one of their major objectives. These hospitals are usually associated with colleges and universities. Besides treating patients, these hospitals provide supervised training for resident psychiatrists and graduate students in the areas of psychology, social work, special education, psychiatric nursing, physical therapy, and other mental health professions. In addition to their teaching, diagnostic, and treatment functions, such hospitals commonly carry on extensive research activities, which are frequently supported by training and/or research grants from governmental agencies, foundations, or other outside sources.

Patients selected for diagnosis and/or treatment in teaching and research hospitals are sometimes chosen because they represent a particular kind of problem that will be of use to the staff for research or demonstration purposes. They may also be selected because they represent a particular geographic area or population designated for treatment in a supporting grant. In any event, patients are usually given a good deal of professional attention as well as thorough and expert care. The mental health professionals-in-training in these institutions are most often very well supervised by senior staff members.

As in other types of mental hospitals, the cost of diagnosis and treatment in teaching and research hospitals varies widely. These institutions usually impose a sliding-fee schedule similar to that used by public mental hospitals.

Entering a Mental Hospital

There are essentially two ways that a person can come to receive diagnostic or treatment services from a mental hospital or residential treatment facility: voluntary admission and involuntary commitment.

Voluntary Admission

A person is voluntarily admitted to a mental hospital when he (or his guardian) more or less freely agrees to seek diagnostic or treatment services from the institution. That decision is often influenced by the intercession of someone else—a family member, friend, family physician, or clergyman. In any event, however, the decision is not made for him by a court or other official body.

A patient admitted voluntarily enters a residential facility under similar circumstances and with prerogatives similar to those enjoyed by an inpatient in a general medical and surgical hospital. While receiving the diagnostic or treatment services he may terminate his residence in the institution and leave, usually after giving advanced written notice. Of course, while he is a resident he agrees to abide by certain rules and procedures established by that particular facility.

Involuntary Commitment

A person is involuntarily committed to a mental hospital when the decision to seek diagnostic or treatment services is made for him by a court or other official body and when that decision is enforced by that court or official body. This element of coercion distinguishes mental health services from the provision of other kinds of human services.

State laws vary considerably regarding the procedures for involuntary commitment to mental institutions. (Detailed information about a specific locality can be obtained from local attorneys, the local probate court, or the state department of mental health.) In general, this is how the process works. First, a petitioner, either a close relative of the patient-to-be or a designated public official, submits a petition to the appropriate court (usually the probate court) alleging that the patient-to-be is in need of immediate psychiatric attention. Usually initiated because the petitioner fears that the patient-to-be may be a danger to himself or to someone else, the allegation charges that the patient is unwilling and/or unable to seek help for himself.

The second step in the involuntary commitment process is the examination of the patient-to-be by (usually) two physicians, who certify that he is in need of inpatient psychiatric treatment. It is important to note that the laws of several states place a time limit on the utility of these certificates.

The final step is the commitment of the patient to the designated institution. After the appropriate court has issued the commitment order, the patient may either surrender himself to the designated mental hospital, or the commitment order will be forcefully executed by the police at the direction of the court.

If an evaluation of the case suggests that the involuntary commitment is to be for an indefinite period of time, the legal proceedings will usually include some safeguards for the protection of the rights of the patient. These safeguards include: (1) giving prior notice of the commitment proceedings to the patient, (2) the provision for a court hearing at which the patient may appear and be represented by a lawyer, and (3) usually, the provision for the patient to be periodically reevaluated in order to determine his need for continuing involuntary hospitalization.

Emergency Involuntary Commitment

Most states have some legal provision for emergency involuntary hospitalization of persons alleged to be in serious and immediate need of psychiatric attention. These procedures allow a citizen to be committed to mental institutions against his will, without a prior hearing or any other chance to defend himself, simply upon certification by a physician that the citizen urgently needs psychiatric help. Often a formal hearing is required within a certain period of time after the emergency commitment order has been executed. Emergency provisions for involuntary hospitalization have important implications for the rights of citizens who are alleged and certified to require psychiatric hospitalization. These provisions vary greatly from state to state and detailed information can be obtained from a lawyer or probate court.

The majority of states with provisions for involuntary commitment also protect the physician who recommended it, even though that recommendation involved an incorrect diagnostic judgment or was later shown to have caused the patient harm or financial loss.

Competence, Commitment, and Civil Rights

An incompetent person is one who (in the opinion of the court) lacks the ability to make the decisions necessary for living in our society. Such a person, by virtue of his official status, usually forfeits a broad range of civil rights enjoyed by his nonincompetent fellow citizens. For example, he may lose the right to dispose of his own money and/or property, to enter into a wide range of contractual agreements including matrimony and divorce, to hold several kinds of licenses including a driver's license, to practice a profession for which he is otherwise qualified, to vote or hold public office, and, of course, he may lose the right of freedom of movement. When a person is involuntarily committed to a mental institution and judged incompetent as a result of that commitment, the court will appoint a guardian to manage his affairs.

Although laws vary considerably from state to state, some states have laws which declare that a person is officially (totally) incompetent when he is committed to a mental institution by virtue of his status as a mental patient, even though the commitment may be involuntary or for diagnostic purposes only. Such laws do not recognize any other areas in which he may be functioning in a normal or even superior manner.

Leaving a Mental Hospital

When an inpatient leaves a mental hospital after diagnosis and/or treatment, an entry explaining *how* he left the premises is made in his official medical record. The exact terminology used to describe the status of a "discharged" patient varies from state to state. In order to illustrate the different official statuses under which a patient can leave a residential mental hospital, three examples of this terminology have been selected for discussion.

Discharge

The word *discharge* has a very special meaning when it applies to leaving a mental hospital. The term refers to a change in the patient's status relative to the institution, both legally and administratively. A patient's being discharged from a mental institution means the mutually-agreed-upon complete termination of the relationship between them. It *does not* mean the same thing as cure, improvement, or any other psychotherapeutic, medical, or educational term.

In the case of readmission to the mental hospital, especially on an involuntary basis, discharged patients are theoretically like any other citizen. That is, if a petition for involuntary commitment to a mental institution were filed with the court against a discharged expatient, that expatient would have at his disposal the same ability and procedures (theoretically) to avoid that hospitalization as the citizen who had not been previously hospitalized.

Convalescent Status

A patient who is released from living in the mental hospital but is still technically a patient is said to be on convalescent status. In theory, convalescent status parallels the medical practice of discharging patients gradually. When this term is applied to patients in mental hospitals, however, it has a very specific meaning. On the positive side, it may be to the patient's advantage to withdraw from inpatient hospitalization in gradual steps. While this process of withdrawal is going on, he may require access to certain services of the hospital such as rehabilitation and medical treatment. Realistically, the patient on convalescent status may be eligible for certain subsidies that he would not qualify for if he were not a patient. These subsidies might cover, for example, payment of room and board for fixed periods of time, payment of tuition and fees for certain schools and job-training programs, and eligibility for certain outpatient medical services.

There are, however, notable disadvantages to withdrawing from a mental hospital under convalescent status. The most important drawback is that the patient is still a patient and, as such, does not always enjoy the full range of civil rights available to nonpatients. For example, the patient on convalescent status may be rehospitalized, even against his will, without the hearing procedure available to other citizens. Thus there are both pros and cons relative to leaving the mental hospital under convalescent status, and the patient, relative, or guardian involved in the procedure should be made aware of them.

Leaving "Against Medical Advice"

Both voluntarily and involuntarily admitted patients occasionally leave the mental hospital without official authorization or permission. This kind of exit from the therapeutic setting is termed *against medical advice*. The term is used primarily as an entry in the record of the patient.

For voluntarily admitted patients, leaving the mental hospital against medical advice is not inherently serious although it does carry a stigma that may make readmission to that hospital somewhat more difficult. Such a notation on a patient's medical record also labels him as being difficult to handle. For involuntarily admitted patients, leaving the mental hospital against medical advice carries more serious implications. It is somewhat analogous to "escaping" or "running away," and if the patient had been admitted under a commitment order, he is, theoretically, a fugitive. The court can direct that such a patient be apprehended and rehospitalized by force, or if necessary the court can direct that the patient be contained in a setting where the security is strict enough to insure his remaining in residence.

Partial Hospitalization

Mental hospital patients are not always hospital residents twenty-four hours of the day. Some patients work during the day in the community and return to the hospital in the evening for psychotherapy, medication, and rest. Under this kind of partial-hospitalization arrangement the mental hospital functions as a carefully planned treatment facility as well as a protected retreat. Another kind of partial hospitalization is called "day care." Day care is not only available for adult patients but is also becoming increasingly common among hospitals and institutions offering children's services. Under this arrangement the patient continues to reside with his family, while going to the hospital in the daytime for psychotherapy, medication, education, vocational training, and so forth. Under the day-care arrangement, the mental hospital functions as a special school and clinic.

Halfway Houses

Halfway houses can be both a partial-hospitalization arrangement and a special living setting for patients on convalescent status. A halfway house is a licensed, supervised residence for patients who are gradually withdrawing from inpatient hospitalization and gradually adjusting to life within the community. It gets its name from the fact that it functions "half-way" between the hospital and the community. Many mental hospitals not only support halfway houses financially, but also provide psychiatric, social work, and psychological services to their staff and residents.

Outpatient Services of Mental Hospitals

It is quite usual for mental hospitals to provide both inpatient and outpatient mental health services. In the broadest sense, outpatient services are those provided to nonresidents of the institution. This area of functioning closely resembles that of clinics discussed in the next section.

The outpatient service of a mental hospital provides three basic levels of service:

1. *Emergency services,* which handle crisis situations. Such crises may or may not require inpatient hospitalization.
2. *Diagnostic services,* which define mental problems. The diagnosed problems may or may not be treated by the inpatient services of the hospital. As a practical matter, diagnostic services also operate quite extensive referral activities because many of the mental disorders they define are more efficiently treated in other settings.
3. *Direct outpatient services,* which support discharged expatients and patients on convalescent status with counseling, rehabilitative

services, continuation of psychotherapy, medication, and somatic treatments. Their general purpose is to ease patients back into the normal life of the community and increase the likelihood of their staying there.

Outpatient departments of mental hospitals often provide mental health services to people who have not been, or are never likely to be, inpatients in the hospital. This aspect of the hospital's functioning most closely resembles a clinic. These services are commonly associated with mental hospitals that have a teaching function or with community mental health centers that are closely associated with the mental hospital.

Mental Hospital Procedures

What happens to a patient when he enters a mental hospital varies considerably from hospital to hospital. There are, however, some fairly standard events in the procedures of most hospitals. These will be discussed in the approximate order in which they occur.

Intake

When a person first presents himself to a mental hospital for inpatient treatment he goes through a series of steps collectively called intake procedures. These are designed to screen the patient and his situation so that the hospital staff can diagnose the problem the patient is presenting and formulate an initial treatment plan. Intake procedures are frequently carried out by a team of mental health professionals who have this as their major responsibility. In many mental hospitals newly admitted patients are temporarily assigned to an intake unit.

Initial diagnosis and intake. The newly admitted patient requires concentrated services that are most efficiently provided in an intake unit. Admission to a mental hospital is somewhat more complicated administratively than admission to a general medical hospital, and matters of guardianship, insurance, and financial arrangements must be dealt with at intake. Initial diagnostic work usually includes a battery of tests and examinations which can be scheduled most efficiently when the patient is available full time on the intake unit. Sound medical reasons also favor segregating newly admitted patients during the intake period.

The most obvious of these is to help control communicable diseases within the hospital. Since patients and staff of most mental hospitals live in fairly close quarters with one another, it is good insurance for the medical staff to be alert for undiagnosed communicable diseases like tuberculosis or hepatitis that the patient might inadvertently bring into the hospital. In addition, certain newly admitted patients may require emergency treatment before any other diagnostic or therapeutic activities can be provided. A common example of such a condition would be an acute psychosis due to drug intoxication.

Temporary ward assignment. A ward in a mental hospital resembles a dormitory more than it does a ward in a general medical and surgical hospital. It is usually made up of dining areas, sleeping areas, educational and recreational areas, a dispensary, nursing stations, staff offices, and administrative areas. It is a complex geographic and social space and in this sense it can be thought of as a community.

A newly admitted patient may be assigned to a special ward for processing and diagnostic work. After this work has been completed he may be transferred to another ward if he is in need of longer hospitalization. As soon as the patient is taken to his ward, a psychiatrist, nurse, or social worker frequently meets with the patient's family in order to explain what the staff and the patient will be doing for the next few days or weeks. Hospital regulations are also explained to the family at this time and a request is made for cooperation in implementing them. In some cases, a descriptive brochure may be handed out.

Restriction of visiting privileges. One of the first disturbing events faced by the family and friends of a newly admitted patient in a mental hospital is the restriction of visiting privileges for a period of time and the suspension of contact between them for the first few days of hospitalization. This kind of regulation is imposed for clinically legitimate reasons, but it is often the cause of bad feelings between the family of the patient and the hospital staff. This resentment can influence their relationship during the course of the patient's hospitalization and also affect the quality of that experience for the patient if due care is not given to interpreting it to the family. In the vast majority of cases, restricting visits with the new patient has nothing to do directly with the family but gives the patient a period of time to settle into the hospital routine with a minimum of interruptions. It also provides the staff with an opportunity to observe this adjustment process. In any case, both the patient and his family should be offered an understandable explanation of the hospital's action. They should also be informed about who is responsible for imposing and removing these restrictions.

Diagnostic "work-ups." Before the staff of the mental hospital can formulate a plan for treating the newly admitted patient, they must first collect a large amount of information about him. This information will concern the patient's physical and emotional condition, social relationships, occupational history, educational achievements, and much more. Of course, it will also contain a detailed history of the patient's mental problem.

A detailed physical examination is usually the first step in the diagnostic process (see chapter 3). The physical usually includes neurological examinations and may involve an EEG and other highly specialized tests. Often the patient is scheduled for a battery of psychological tests early in the process. The psychiatrist and the social worker may also spend several hours interviewing the patient during this period.

One of the most important sources of information about the new patient during the diagnostic process is provided by the skilled observations of the nursing staff and the ward attendants. As the information is gathered, the whole staff meets to share their observations and exchange ideas related to the formulation of the patient's evolving treatment plan. It is not uncommon for the patient to be invited to at least a portion of such meetings so that he may clarify particular questions raised by staff members. He may also be given an opportunity to address any questions he may have to various members of the hospital staff.

It is also not unusual, especially in state and teaching hospitals, for outside consultants to be called in during the various steps of the intake process, including the diagnostic conferences. The product of all this information gathering and information sharing is the development of a workable treatment plan designed specifically for this new patient.

Treatment

After the newly admitted patient has gone through the intake phase of his stay in the mental hospital, he will sometimes be transferred to a treatment unit (or ward). Life in a treatment unit is much different from that in an intake unit. Ideally, the treatment ward should function as a therapeutic community for the patients who reside there. Treatment during this phase is designed to modify the patient's behavior in such a way that he becomes able to resume his life in the wider community outside of the mental hospital.

The daily routine of the average patient in the average mental hospital treatment unit would be impossible to describe because the needs and hospital routines of each patient vary so widely. Nonetheless, some activities will be described in which the average patient would likely be involved. A given patient might participate in some, all, or none of these activities, depending on his particular situation and that of the hospital in which he is being treated.

Assignment of a therapist. The responsibility for each newly admitted patient is always assigned to a professional member of the hospital staff. This staff member is usually a resident psychiatrist. In large state hospitals with chronic manpower shortages, the ratio of psychiatrists to patients may be such that the individual patient may not have the opportunity for frequent consultations with the psychiatrist. In such cases the treatment and progress of patients may be coordinated and monitored by other staff members. In any event, always some individual (with a name and a title) is responsible for each patient in the institution.

The therapist is the person who administers, coordinates, and monitors the major part of the patient's treatment. As the official link between the patient and the hospital, the therapist is responsible for knowing as much as possible about the patient, his situation, and his progress. In addition, he is responsible for the compilation of the entries in the patient's records. He authorizes leaves from the hospital and sees to other administrative matters that bear upon the patient's treatment. One of the therapist's most important duties is to coordinate and preside at the various staff conferences dealing with his patient. Besides serving as a resource person for the other staff members in matters concerning his patient, he continuously monitors the patient's progress. Finally, he assumes responsibility for changes in his patient's treatment plan and for all other major decisions, including discharge, that will affect his patient.

Medications. Patients in mental hospitals are frequently given medications which are prescribed for them as part of their treatment plan. These medications are most often distributed to the patients by the unit nurses near the meal hours. Usually the patients report in a group to the nursing station, a procedure that may look like a semimilitary operation but which is done this way for legitimate reasons: it facilitates the dispensing of the medications; it allows the nurse to observe the patient taking the medicine; it aids in making the proper entry into the patient's medical record; and most important, it helps to eliminate distribution errors.

Rest and relaxation.   Most mental hospital routines include periods of rest and relaxation, usually after meals. During these times the patients may retire to the day room of their unit to talk, smoke, play cards, watch television, or just to rest. If a patient has grounds privileges, he is usually free to wander about the hospital grounds.

Recreation therapy.   Because appropriate recreation is such a prominent part of a satisfactory everyday life and because so many patients have experienced difficulty in this area of their lives, many mental hospitals have established programs of recreation therapy. Through carefully planned individual and group recreation activities, professionally trained recreation therapists help the patients discover new and satisfying ways of occupying their leisure time. The recreation therapist is an important member of the mental health team of the hospital because recreational activities are particularly appealing events for integrating the patient into the therapeutic community of the treatment unit. These events are frequently the first structured activities in which the patient is able to participate. Consequently, part of the average patient's day is often spent in individual or group recreational activities supervised by the recreation therapist.

Drinking and smoking.   With possible rare exception, mental hospitals prohibit the possession or use of alcoholic beverages by patients. This is done for several reasons. First, many patients have had problems with the use of alcohol. Second, since most mental hospitals are either licensed or operated by state governments, enforced state regulations prohibit the use of alcoholic beverages on the premises (by anyone). And, finally, alcohol does not "mix well" with many of the drugs that are prescribed in the treatment of patients.

Most mental hospitals permit patients to smoke in certain designated areas and on the grounds. Restrictions are applied to smoking in certain working and sleeping areas for reasons of safety.

Patients and hospital work. Constructive work is one of the most important activities of anyone in our society, and in some mental hospitals patients are encouraged to perform regularly assigned tasks (or work duties) around the hospital. In many cases, the patients so employed are paid for their efforts, which might include clerical and messenger duties or work on buildings and grounds or in the kitchen, gift shop, and cafeteria. If a patient has some skill or trade, the hospital endeavors to make use of it as part of the treatment plan. Electricians, typists, switchboard operators, and chefs, for example, may be able to practice their skills on a part-time basis while they are inpatients.

Occupational therapy. Many mental hospitals have extensive programs designed to help patients develop new occupational skills or to strengthen those already developed. Many patients therefore spend a significant portion of their time engaged in these activities under the guidance of the professionally trained occupational therapists on the hospital's staff. Since the ability to work satisfactorily is an essential aspect of life in our culture, the occupational therapist is a key member of the treatment team of the progressive mental hospital.

Educational programs. Fully accredited high school programs are included in the therapeutic programs of many mental hospitals, and school-related activities may occupy a large portion of the average day, especially in the case of younger patients. These schools are staffed by professionally trained special education teachers. The skill and training of these teachers, as well as their option to design individual programs for each of their patient-students, account for the fact that many hospital schools are educationally equivalent to public school programs. Provision for the formal education of young people who are inpatients in mental institutions is a vital part of the hospital's therapeutic program. It is not at all unusual for hospitals with these educational programs to have a class or two graduate each year with fully accredited high school diplomas.

Intramural activities. Unit athletic teams and special-interest clubs (like garden clubs and photography clubs) are available in many mental hospitals. Patients are encouraged to spend a portion of their time developing new interests or renewing previous pastimes represented by these clubs.

One of the most important of the intramural activities in some hospitals is the patient council, a form of representative government for the patients. Elected patient-representatives from each unit meet on a regular basis to plan projects of mutual interest, to formulate and review certain rules, and to conduct similar business. Like other activities in a well-designed therapeutic program, participation in self-governing programs has behind it a rehabilitative rationale, which is to prepare the patient for responsible citizenship outside the hospital. A newsletter and various other publications are typical products of an active patient council.

Religion and pastoral counseling. Most mental hospitals have chaplains on the staff to look after the religious needs of the patients and to provide pastoral counseling as appropriate. Those patients who profess an active religious faith are able to spend a portion of each day or week in worship and other activities of their religious faith.

Individual psychotherapy. Not all patients in mental hospitals are engaged in individual psychotherapy, but when it is prescribed as part of the patient's treatment plan, anywhere from an hour a week to an hour a day may be spent in regularly scheduled sessions. The psychotherapist who meets with the patient in such sessions is usually the coordinator of the patient's treatment plan.

Group psychotherapy. It is not uncommon for a large percentage of patients in a mental hospital to be involved in group psychotherapy. Depending on the details of a patient's treatment plan, it is less common for him to be involved in *both* individual and group psychotherapy. Like individual psychotherapy, group therapy is usually scheduled on a regular basis. Patients involved in it will therefore spend a portion of each day or week in "group."

Case conferences. Case conferences are formal meetings of the entire unit staff, scheduled for the purposes of exchanging information and making decisions about the treatment of particular patients. Because these are the primary decision-making meetings concerning the patient, administrators, outside professionals, and appropriate consultants may also be included. In some hospitals the patient and his fam-

.

ily are included as well. If the patient or his family has engaged the services of an outside professional person (a professional advocate) to monitor the patient's progress in the hospital, he is included in these conferences. Although case conferences are not part of the patient's hospital routine, they should be a periodic and regular component of his inpatient experience in an indirect way.

Evaluation

Interest is growing across the country in proposals to require state institutions to periodically review each patient in their care. Massachusetts, for example, recently passed a law not only requiring all state institutions to periodically review each patient, but also to make available to the patient and his guardian the results of the review process, including a record of all treatments administered and responses to those treatments, a statement of the need for further hospitalization, and a list of alternatives to institutionalization that have been explored by the staff. In addition to making the operations of state mental hospitals more answerable to the needs of their clients, such laws should also serve to shorten the period of residential treatment and to emphasize the use of nonresidential treatment alternatives wherever possible.

CHAPTER 6

Mental Health Clinics: Outpatient Treatment Facilities

A mental health clinic is a professional organization that offers some kind of mental health service (advice, counseling, diagnosis, or treatment) in an outpatient setting. Although the word *clinic* has definite medical implications, it is more a concept than a location in the "mental health" sense. Just what kind of advice, counseling, or treatment is given to whom by which professional persons varies greatly from clinic to clinic, as does the range or scope of the services offered.

Since mental health clinics are usually outpatient (or nonresidential) facilities, clients or patients use them as they would the office of a private physician. They go to the clinic periodically to receive a unit of service and then they return to their homes and regular community routines. The encounter with the mental health clinic is brief, lasting from thirty minutes to a few hours at most per visit. In some cases, the services of the mental health clinic are brought to the client, but even then the time requirements and the client's living arrangements are about the same. There are, however, a few limited exceptions to this generalization, the most common of which is the court clinic. Here, a very specialized kind of mental health service is provided to individuals who have come to the attention of the law (see the relevant discussions in chapter 9).

Although patients are not committed to clinics as they are to mental hospitals, they may be subject to accepting mental health services from clinics under official pressure in certain circumstances. For example, a court could impose the acceptance of clinical diagnostic or treatment services as a condition of probation or in connection with divorce, domestic relations, or adoption cases.

69

Many social agencies function very much like mental health clinics. These agencies are usually staffed by professionally trained social workers and supervised, student social workers. There is a trend now to to include paraprofessionals or community health workers on the staff who serve to bridge the gap between those who give professional services and the clients of the agency.

Social agencies are usually equipped to deal with a broad range of mental problems including diagnosis, treatment, referral, and follow-up. Some social agencies employ psychiatrists or other physicians to provide specific medical services on a part-time, consulting, or contractual basis. Thus, when a client presents a problem requiring the attention of a physician, such as the prescription of medication or the administration of somatic therapy, he might be referred to the appropriate practitioner.

Licensing and Accreditation

Usually the state government, through the State Department of Mental Health or another designated governmental agency, monitors the activities of mental health clinics. Official sanction is required in order to participate in subsidies both from the government and from community funds and to be eligible to receive certain kinds of grants. When a mental health clinic is involved in the training of professional persons, a specific accreditation has to be obtained from the organizations representing that particular field of training. The American Psychological Association and the National Association of Social Workers are examples of organizations which provide accreditation.

Classification

Like residential treatment facilities, mental health clinics can be classified in any number of ways. Three of these ways are: (1) by funding sources and sponsorship (private, public, and teaching and research), (2) by the services provided by the clinic, and (3) by the population served by the clinic.

Funding Sources and Sponsorship

Mental health clinics can be supported with either private or public funds or both. The sponsorship of a particular mental health clinic is important because it may influence both a client's eligibility to receive services and the cost of those services.

Private clinics. Private mental health clinics are the outpatient counterparts of private mental hospitals, although sometimes these too are known as "clinics." The outpatient clinics offer mental health services on a fee-for-service basis, and their financial support comes mainly from fees collected from the clients they serve. The mental health services offered by these private clinics may be very broad indeed. In addition to offering direct services to patients, such clinics may, in certain circumstances, also offer consultation to professional persons, agencies, institutions, and groups within the community on a contractual basis. It is not unusual for such clinics to employ psychologists, psychiatrists, social workers, and other mental health professionals and to use these people in teams, much as the comprehensive public facilities do.

Some private mental health clinics operate like group psychiatric practices and may be composed of a partnership of mental health professionals who accept patients for diagnosis and treatment in the same way that a single private practitioner would. A clinic may be independent or function as part of a larger complex of facilities such as a private general hospital or a private psychiatric institute.

A new and developing trend in the operation of private mental health clinics involves a contractual arrangement between a group of mental health professionals and a unit of government or industry. Under such an arrangement the unit of government buys a large block of mental health services for distribution to some group of citizens or employees. This kind of arrangement is quite different from the usual public mental health facilities because under it the government buys private services in the open market and makes them available to citizens rather than providing the services as a direct function of the government. The arrangement is similar to public mental health services in that the government frequently subsidizes the cost of the service that the consumer receives.

Public clinics. Public mental health clinics, the outpatient counterparts of public mental hospitals, offer nonresidential services to the general population of some geographic area like a neighborhood, town, or county. The professionals who provide the services offered by these clinics are usually public employees. Although such clinics may collect payment on a sliding-fee schedule, they are supported and, if need be, subsidized by public funds. Almost every level of government, from federal to city, can and does support mental health clinics.

The kinds of public mental health clinic services offered by governments vary widely—from emergency-room services of city hospitals, to county child guidance clinics, to federally funded community mental health centers serving populations of up to 200,000 people. Because mental health clinics are more a concept of nonresidential service delivery than a location or a set of offices, both the clinic's method of operation and its physical facilities vary widely. A clinic may be housed in a single facility, or part of a larger institution such as a city hospital, or composed of a series of outposts.

A growing direction in the delivery of mental health services is the movement of mental health professionals out of clinic buildings and into the communities they serve, bringing services to the clients rather than having the clients come to a place where the services are dispensed during office hours. Mental health professionals are beginning to realize that intervention in psychological problems must be available on a round-the-clock basis. This approach has a number of advantages: it offers the possibility of earlier intervention, which could mean the deterrence of future treatment lasting longer and costing more; and it promises to make mental health services available to people who might not otherwise seek them in more structured and formal clinic settings.

Teaching and research clinics. Teaching and research facilities, like those associated with universities, also operate mental health clinics. These clinics are the outpatient counterparts of teaching and research mental hospitals and are similar in operation, eligibility for service, and fees for treatment.

Like other mental health clinics, clinics associated with teaching and research facilities concentrate a good deal of their energies on diagnosis and, where appropriate, on making treatment referrals to other units within the academic setting or to other agencies or treatment facilities within the community. Because the staffs of these clinics usually include a number of well-supervised graduate students studying the various mental health professions, clients often receive an extra measure of sophisticated attention.

Some Services of Mental Health Clinics

One of the best ways to describe mental health clinics is in terms of the services they provide. Although some mental health clinics offer a specialized type of mental health service, most of them are now beginning to offer a wide range of comprehensive services. This trend characterizes all kinds of clinics—private, public, and teaching and research.

Emergency services. Many mental health clinics operate twenty-four-hour walk-in or telephone services for mental health emergencies. Such an emergency can be broadly defined as a situation in which a person is at the verge of, or going through, a severe psychological disorganization and as a result may be on the point of endangering either himself or someone else.

The concept of emergency services (aside from emergency-room treatment provided by general hospitals) is relatively new in the field of mental health practice. Emergency services have been a bit late in becoming established because, to many people including professionals, mental problems have been considered conditions that develop only after a long period of time. In addition, other community agents like the police and the clergy were traditionally called upon to deal with them. Finally, the trend toward emergency services gained impetus when the Mental Retardation Facilities and Community Mental Health Centers and Construction Act of 1963 made it mandatory for all federally funded community mental health centers to provide these services.

A walk-in emergency service as part of a mental health clinic is open and staffed twenty-four hours a day, seven days a week. Clients may walk in at any time of the day or night and receive immediate service. The staff of the walk-in clinic diagnoses the presented problem and, where appropriate, begins to implement a plan of treatment immediately. The treatment may involve the prescription of medication, short-term psychotherapy, referral to another mental hospital or mental health service facility, or even emergency commitment to a mental hospital. Some mental health clinics provide facilities for emergency short-term hospitalization as a supplement to their other emergency services, or simply act as "troubleshooting" clinics. Many clinics operate a twenty-four-hour emergency telephone service manned by highly skilled mental health workers. The twenty-four-hour "hot line" is a very important service because, in those communities where such a system is in operation, no person with a mental problem is more than a few steps or minutes away from timely mental health information and help.

Although the hot line offers the general possibility of vastly expanding the services of the mental health clinic, there are two kinds of problems in particular to which it is almost perfectly suited. First, the person who may be thinking of taking his own life has a dedicated, skilled, and understanding friend available to him when he picks up the telephone. He does not even have to dial the number; he need only ask the operator to connect him with the hot line of the mental health clinic. Second, in addition to being timely, emergency phone service offers the assurance that the exchange will be confidential and that the caller may, if he wishes, remain anonymous. This feature of emergency telephone services seems to have particular appeal for young people, especially those calling for information or assistance with drug-related problems. There is never a charge for these services.

Diagnostic services. Like the intake section of a mental hospital, most mental health clinics provide extensive diagnostic services, which often include a full range of psychiatric, neurological, and general medical examinations as well as psychological and social work services. The diagnostic information gathered by the staff of the clinic is usually compiled by a diagnostic team which defines the problem and then makes recommendations for treatment. This treatment may be carried out at the clinic itself or a referral may be made to some other mental health facility. In the case of court clinics, the recommendations of the diagnostic team often take the form of professional opinions to be considered by a judge in making decisions about a legal proceeding in which the patient is involved.

Treatment services. The treatment services of mental health clinics are similar to those offered by mental hospitals and include the prescription of medication, the administration of various kinds of somatic therapy, group psychotherapy, individual psychotherapy, and family counseling and therapy. The client of the mental health clinic is usually assigned a therapist who is responsible for the implementation of the client's treatment plan.

Mental health clinics do not usually offer the same range of treatment that progressive mental hospitals do, such as recreational or occupational therapy and pastoral counseling. If these services are required as part of the treatment plan, the client may be referred to another agency or organization.

Referral and coordination services. Because mental health clinics are frequently the first formal agencies approached by persons seeking help, their staff members usually devote a good deal of effort to screening, diagnostic, and referral activities. In this respect the mental health clinics often serve as "clearinghouses" which direct people to more specialized but less publicly visible treatment facilities that may exist within the community.

Certain treatment plans may require the involvement of two or more specialized agencies; thus, the referring mental health clinic often furnishes the services necessary to coordinate these initial treatment efforts. Coordination of mental health services is also one of the most important functions of comprehensive community mental health centers.

Services for Special Populations

Another way of classifying mental health clinics is in terms of special populations with which they are particularly well equipped to deal. Some such populations are: children (served by child guidance clinics); married couples (marriage counseling clinics); persons with drug-related problems (drug counseling clinics, "street clinics," and methadone maintenance clinics); persons with alcohol-related problems (alcohol abuse clinics, antibuse clinics); senior citizen clinics (geriatric clinics); or persons with seriously limited intellectual ability (mental retardation clinics).

Some mental health clinics specialize in providing services for groups of people with something in common, such as membership in a church or other organization, or residency in a particular neighborhood or geographic area. The population grouping might also be based on such commonly held past experiences as serving in the military or working in an industry or unit of government.

In addition, certain clinics expend a good deal of their resources providing consultation services to other mental health care givers, including social agencies, family physicians, teachers, clergymen, and police officers. This "consultation and education" function is a required activity of all federally funded comprehensive community mental health centers.

Contacting Mental Health Clinics

A person may begin a treatment relationship with a mental health clinic in several ways. He may be referred to the clinic as a result of an earlier contact with the emergency service of a general hospital or with a twenty-four-hour telephone emergency service, or he may simply walk into the clinic unannounced seeking help with a mental problem. In fact, a large percentage of clients come to the clinic on their own initiative. Some people come because they were referred by a family physician, clergyman, teacher, or even a concerned relative or friend. Others become clients because it has been stipulated as a condition of probation, domestic relations, or other legal proceeding in which they are involved.

Clients of mental health clinics are not committed to the clinic in the way a patient may be committed to a mental hospital. As a rule, they come to receive mental health services and, having received them, are more or less free to terminate their relationship with the clinic whenever they choose. The client of the mental health clinic can expect the same kind of confidential relationship with the clinic staff that the patients in residential facilities or those under the care of private therapists have a right to enjoy.

Cost of Services

The fees charged by mental health clinics are similar to those described for mental hospitals (see chapter 5). Private clinics, for example, charge on a fee-for-service basis. As in the case of residential facilities, the patient of a private mental health clinic is usually billed for each unit of service he receives. For example, individual psychotherapy would be billed at rates approximating twenty to forty dollars per hour. Medications and other medical services are usually billed as they would be by a private medical practitioner. Public mental health clinics frequently bill for their services according to a sliding-fee schedule in which those with higher incomes pay relatively more and those with lower incomes pay relatively less. Since units of government fund the operation of public mental health clinics, the cost of their services to the consumer is usually less than in nonfunded private facilities. This also holds true for facilities subsidized by the United Fund and certain other philanthropic interests.

When mental health clinics impose a charge for all or part of their services and when the client is directly responsible for making the payment, the client may be required to pay each time he visits the clinic. Some clinics issue statements for all services rendered during a particular time period, like a week or month. Some mental health clinics, like private psychotherapists, reserve a weekly portion of time for each client. Clinics following this policy often bill the client for each session whether the client actually comes to the clinic or not, unless he gives advanced notice that he will not be there on a certain day.

One of the first things a consumer of mental health services should do when he contacts a mental health clinic is to inquire about the cost of services. This information will be needed in order to negotiate an adequate therapeutic contract with the clinic.

Subsidizing the Cost of Services

In many cases, the clients of mental health clinics can receive outside help in paying for all or part of the service obtained from the clinic. The most obvious subsidy is represented by the government's direct support of certain mental health clinics.

Some prepaid group insurance plans have provisions for reimbursing policy holders for a fixed amount of mental health services obtained through a clinic. Other prepaid insurance arrangements actually provide the necessary services directly to members or subscribers. Certain health insurance contracts offer payment for a stated number of visits and/or service units. Such contracts should be checked to see if they will provide such assistance.

Persons eligible for public welfare or public assistance are often entitled to financial help with the costs involved in receiving mental health clinic services. In some circumstances veterans can claim clinical services at reduced fees. (Mental health care may also be available to the veteran directly through the outpatient departments of the various U.S. Veterans Administration Hospitals.) Members of certain labor unions and employees of some organizations are also eligible to receive mental health clinic services provided at reduced or no cost by their sponsoring organization. Persons who are eligible for medicare services may also be entitled to receive mental health clinic care, subject to some limits.

Most mental health clinics employ social workers who are trained to advise clients about the subsidies for which they may be eligible. These social workers can also assist the client in making the proper arrangements to obtain any financial help.

Intake

The intake phase of a mental health clinic's operations, functionally similar to that employed by mental hospitals, involves the careful screening of the presented complaint to determine whether or not it is a problem that can be handled by the clinic's treatment staff. The intake phase also includes a good deal of administrative work with the new client. This activity is concerned with determining if the new client is eligible for the services offered by the clinic as well as making arrangements for payment. Generally speaking, clinics do more screening, initial diagnosis, and referral work than does the average hospital.

In making an appraisal or diagnosis of the patient's problem and the formulation of an appropriate treatment plan, the staff may take three broad courses of action:

1. If the presented problem is not really a mental disorder, the client is informed of the finding, and the relationship between the client and the clinic usually terminates. It is very important to remember that

the diagnostic process frequently results in finding no psychological problem. Not everyone who thinks he has a mental problem does, in fact, have one. The converse of this statement is also unfortunately true. Some people do not consider drug addiction, alcoholism, and certain socially defined delinquent activities the results of psychological impairments, but consider them normal or natural aspects of their way of living.

2. The diagnostic activity of the clinic may reveal that the new client has a mental problem of a type that would not be best treated by the clinic that diagnosed it. In such cases, the client is referred to a mental health facility better equipped to treat that particular problem. Similarly, if it is revealed that the new client has another kind of problem—perhaps medical, legal, economic, or educational—the client is referred to the institution, facility, or professional person who will be able to help him.

3. If the problem is solvable by the clinic itself, the new client is transferred to the treatment staff of the clinic. At this point a therapeutic contract is negotiated between the client and the staff of the clinic.

Treatment

Mental health clinics generally employ the same kinds of treatment that are offered by progressive mental hospitals, and the client usually comes to the clinic on a regularly scheduled basis to participate in his treatment. Most often this involves an appointment of about an hour once or twice each week. These arrangements vary widely depending upon the client's situation, the treatment that has been prescribed, and the operating mode of the individual clinic.

Clients use the services of mental health clinics the way they use the services of a physician, a marriage counselor, or an educational tutor. That is, between visits they go about their usual business in the community. Because clients spend only a few hours a week at the clinic, most clinics allow some flexibility in the scheduling of appointments. They frequently make their services available during evening or nonbusiness hours so that clients will not have to disrupt their occupational schedules unnecessarily. This is particularly important for married couples, families, or other groups of persons receiving treatment together.

Clients of mental health clinics usually have a therapist who is responsible for formulating and implementing the treatment plan—a nurse, social worker, psychiatrist, or other professional. The mental health worker monitors the client's progress, updates the treatment plan when necessary, and coordinates the activities of other clinic staff members involved with his client. Together with the client, he then sets goals for the course of treatment and determines with the client when those goals have been met and when the therapy is to terminate.

Terminating the Relationship

At the very beginning of their treatment relationship, the most important thing a client and a therapist do together is to negotiate an explicit therapeutic contract, which states the goals of the treatment as well as the responsibilities of the client and the therapist in achieving them. As the course of the treatment proceeds, the client and the therapist should make it a point to review their progress periodically. They may update and modify the contract as they go along, as long as they both agree to each new provision. Ideally, the therapeutic relationship should be terminated by mutual agreement when the goals of the treatment specified in the contract have been reached. It is important to note that the termination of the therapeutic relationship is a step-by-step process that begins with the negotiation of the contract and continues as a series of concrete and reachable goals throughout the course of the treatment. Termination should never be sudden or come as a surprise to either the client or the therapist.

Sometimes the client and the therapist are unable to reach the goals specified in the contract. When this happens, even after both parties have explored all the available alternatives, termination and/or referral to another agency or practitioner might be considered.

Even with adequate therapeutic contracts, dropouts from treatment are not infrequent. After all, no therapist can be expected to solve all the mental disorders presented to him. Moreover, some problems are simply not solvable with the resources available for the task.

Discharge

When the relationship between a client and a mental health clinic terminates, the clinic simply "closes the case" and the client stops coming to his regularly scheduled appointments. If the client is referred to another agency as a part of the termination procedure, he begins another relationship and negotiates a new therapeutic contract with the new agency.

When a client wants information pertaining to his diagnosis and treatment relayed to another agency, he must sign a written form for the release of that information. In some instances, a therapist could consider that the release of certain data might be harmful to the well-being of the patient. The therapist may thus elect to withhold that information even though the patient has authorized its release. An example of such a potentially harmful bit of information might be the inclusion in the client's case record of a formal diagnosis (like schizophrenia or character disorder) which might become a stigma to the patient long after therapy is terminated.

Since utilization of the services of mental health clinics does not usually involve the client's competence, involuntary commitment, or forfeiture of civil rights, the termination transaction is normally an internal bookkeeping activity of the clinic's records section. If the relationship with the clinic has been ordered as a result of a court action (like a condition of probation or in connection with a domestic relations case) pertinent information about the diagnosis or the course of treatment may be made available to the court by means of professional conferences and/or written reports.

CHAPTER 7

Mental Health Treatment Programs in the Schools

Special Education Classes

The public schools of the nation operate a vast network of mental health diagnostic and treatment facilities. This network includes a number of separate elements, many of which are found in large or moderately large school systems. The programs are usually operated and coordinated by the special education or special services department of the school system.

The most formal of the special education programs are the special education classes, which are designed to meet the educational needs of a group of students with a behavior or learning problem in common. These classes are usually categorized according to the particular behavior problem or learning difficulty with which they primarily deal. School systems with special education departments normally offer two or more special classes for children who are physically or visually handicapped, mentally retarded (now called a developmental disability), emotionally disturbed, or perceptually handicapped. The uniformity of these programs from school system to school system is due in large part to the active participation of state governments which subsidize and regulate their operation. State governments both certify the diagnosticians who screen students for admission and set requirements for training the personnel who teach in the various programs.

Admission

To be eligible for admission to a special education class, a student must be examined by a state-certified school psychologist or diagnostician. In some areas, school systems entertain recommendations for special class placements from other professional practitioners like psychologists, psychiatrists, or physicians who are not directly employed by the school system.

In its purest form, the special education class is composed of a small group of students who have some particular educational or social need in common. The teacher is usually a trained professional whose specialty is dealing with the exceptional requirements of his class. These teachers supplement their skills, training, and sensitivity with specially designed teaching materials and innovative teaching techniques. They usually do have access to professional consultation from other teachers and educational specialists working within the school system.

State Board of Education Regulations

State boards of education (or public instruction) furnish copies of the regulations governing the admission of students to special classes, maximum class size, teacher qualifications, and so forth. These regulations spell out the need for parental permission for the enrollment of students in these classes and the intervals at which enrolled students must be reevaluated. They also describe alternate ways of obtaining treatment and diagnostic services through the school system, information that could be of great practical importance if efforts to obtain service are frustrated by long waiting lists or the absence of places in existing special education programs.

Special Classes for Students with Developmental Disabilities

According to recent federal legislation, developmental disabilities are conditions which occur before the age of eighteen years and subsequently impair some area of an individual's functioning. Usually, these conditions are associated with some neurological or physical deficit. Mental retardation is a broad category of functional deficits that are included as developmental disabilities. In addition, mental retardation is a category of learning problems dealt with by special education programs in the schools.

Special classes for mentally retarded children provide formal instruction for students who cannot keep up with the pace in regular classes.

Students become eligible for placement in special classes for "slow learners" by virtue of their performance on standardized tests on intellectual ability. These tests are administered and the results interpreted by certified diagnosticians. Students are referred for testing by classroom teachers on the basis of the student's past and/or present performance in the class. Classes for mentally retarded students are sometimes divided into "tracks" based on the intellectual capacity of students assigned to them.

Educable classes. Educable classes are designed for students whose intellectual capacities are such that they can avail themselves of formal education within the school system. In order to accomplish this, however, teaching methods and instructional materials are modified to fit their slower pace of learning. The primary requirement for a student's admission to such a class is that he be administered a standardized intelligence test and that his score be within the range stipulated in the state regulations. The requires scores vary from area to area; information about local standards may be obtained from the appropriate state department of education.

Trainable classes. The intellectual capacities of some students are limited to the point that they are not able to master formal academic material even in special classes. Some of these students, however, can be taught to pursue occupations in line with their abilities. These students are sometimes referred to as "trainable." The programs and materials used in trainable classes are intended to prepare these individuals to live as independently as possible after their formal education is completed. The requirements for placement in classes for trainable students includes an earned score on a standardized intelligence test as stipulated in the state department of education regulations.

Special Classes for Emotionally Disturbed Students

The term *emotional disturbance* is a concept or an opinion about the cause of some particular behavior or group of behaviors. Its presence is inferred by a teacher or diagnostician on the basis of some observable behavior. Some such signs of emotional disturbance might be overactivity, listlessness, chronic inattention, fearfulness, social immaturity, or inability to play appropriately with other children. More severe signs of emotional disturbance would be cruelty to younger children or animals, fire-setting, stealing, or self-destructive behavior. The potential length of such a list is long, indeed.

Many students who are classified as having emotional disturbances have normal or even superior intellectual capacities. Special education classes for these students often concentrate on the development of interpersonal and social skills as well as on the mastery of academic material.

Special Classes for Minimally Brain-damaged Students

Children may show many problematic behaviors that are assumed to be caused by subtle kinds of brain damage. Although this group of problematic behaviors is frequently referred to as *"minimal brain damage"* (MBD), there are well over thirty diagnostic labels applied to the same general condition. The labels of this group most often used in school systems are "hyperactive" and "perceptually handicapped."

Two aspects of the classification minimal brain damage are important and deserve the attention of parents. First, the fact that there are over thirty labels applied to it indicates that none of these labels is as specific as it might ideally be. Second, it is likely that future research will show that what we now call minimal brain damage or "perceptual handicap" is really several different and separate problematic behaviors with several different, but perhaps related, causes. If this possibility should materialize, a number of diversified treatments for these various conditions will likely evolve. Each such label should then be viewed with suspicion and students to whom these labels are applied should be treated as individuals rather than as members of a diagnostic class.

Students who are said to be perceptually handicapped are assumed to have difficulty interpreting (with their brains) what their eyes see. These students often come to the attention of the schools because they have great difficulty with the mechanics of reading. They are frequently inattentive, overactive, and accident-prone as well.

Special education classes for minimally brain-damaged students are often arranged so as to minimize distractions and to maximize the focusing of attention upon the material being presented. These arrangements may include semiprivate cubicles for study and work. Bright colors, patterns, and posters may be conspicuously absent in these areas. Work assignments may be presented in the form of concrete, step-by-step programmed instructions.

Some researchers believe that certain minimally brain-damaged children will outgrow their learning handicap as they mature physically, usually by about eighteen years of age. They believe that the main responsibility of special education for these students is to keep them from falling behind so that when they mature they will be ready for normal living and learning. As with emotional disturbances, MBD and perceptual handicaps do not seem to be related to intellectual capacities and many students having such handicaps exhibit normal and even superior intellectual abilities.

Since any of the diagnoses of various behaviors that are presumed to be caused by minimal brain damage imply the existence of a neurological condition, a tentative diagnosis should be confirmed by a neurologist in every case. When such a condition is suspected, parents should have the diagnosis confirmed before the student is labeled and assigned to a special class. The neurologist can be of great help to students, parents, and teachers in several ways:

1. The signs of MBD are very similar to those of other behavior disorders; thus it is often quite difficult to differentiate MBD from other conditions, especially in younger children. In every suspected case the neurologist should be called upon to rule it out.
2. The neurologist's findings, together with those of the teacher and the psychologist, provide valuable information for planning and evaluating individual education programs.
3. In some cases the neurologist can prescribe medication which will enable the student to function quite normally in the regular classroom. Such a treatment plan, if successful, can eliminate the necessity for special class placement altogether and thereby guarantee a more normal intellectual and social development for the student.

Some Comments on Special Education Classes

In cases where school authorities are contemplating a testing referral for placement in a special class, regulations often require that advanced written notice be given to the student's parents or guardian. In addition, regulations usually require written permission from parents or guardian before the testing can proceed. Advanced notice and written permission are important public protections and parents faced with this situation should be aware of them and use them intelligently. Once a student has been formally labeled "a problem" he may well have difficulty overcoming the label in the future. Since labels like "emotionally disturbed" or "hyperactive" are inherently negative, the child who carries such a label may find that he has a "reputation" which follows him from year to year in school.

That teachers may have quite different expectations of a labeled student than they have of one not labeled is another factor to consider. This is an important factor because the reaction of the teacher to the student and his label may be such that the quality of the student's educational experience is altered long after he leaves the special education classroom. Placement of a student in a special education class is, in many cases, a wise decision made in the student's best interest. On the other hand, a special class placement can have undesirable long-range consequences. Such a decision should be made only after all other alternatives have been explored and exhausted.

If a parent is advised that a special class placement is being contemplated for his child, he should engage the services of appropriate professional counsel from outside the school system. It is a good idea for parents to have this additional and independent source of information when they are faced with making such an important decision about the life of their child. A wise decision requires confirming the diagnosis reached by the school employees as well as a thorough exploration of treatment possibilities available both within and outside of the school system.

Tutors and Mental Health Programs in the Schools

The placement of students in special education classes has many positive aspects to recommend it. There are, however, some notable disadvantages to the segregation of behaviorally classified students in isolated special classes. Perhaps the most noteworthy of these disadvantages is the usual separation of the special class student from the mainstream of life in his school. Those students with some particular behavioral problem who have developed normal or superior levels of competence in other school-related areas of their lives may more profitably be assisted by special programs which address themselves *solely* to the area in which the student is having his difficulty. This individualized approach to special education has the advantage of avoiding the isolation of special classes by offering special help only where it is needed and by permitting the student to avail himself of the other normal school activities.

A tutorial experience is a program designed to assist an individual student with a specific area of academic or behavioral difficulty. It is important to note that tutorial assistance in public schools can be applied to the remediation of academic deficiencies as well as to the development of competence or excellence.

Some progressive public school systems have eliminated the more traditional segregated special education classes from their academic programs and have begun to deal with the specific learning difficulties of former special-class students with individually tailored tutorial programs. The teachers and administrators of these school systems feel that the academic and social difficulties of individual students can best be remedied by expert individual attention. Their action in eliminating segregated special education classrooms indicates that they believe the cost of blanket isolation in special classes to be greater than the benefits.

Crisis Intervention Services in the Schools

Some school systems employ specifically trained *crisis teachers* to resolve behavioral and emotional crises of children. These teachers function as specialized troubleshooters who minimize classroom disruptions and maximize the amount of time that potentially disruptive students spend in regular classes and activities. Crisis teachers have often had extra training in counseling, special education, or school psychology.

Social Work in the Schools

Some schools employ professional social workers who serve to bridge the gaps between individual students, the school, and the community. School social workers also see some students in individual supportive psychotherapy. School systems employing social workers or other psychotherapists usually have regulations prohibiting the beginning of a therapeutic relationship without the written consent of the student's parent or guardian. In this context, a therapeutic relationship is sometimes defined as more than a certain number (usually two or three) of regularly scheduled appointments between the social worker and the student.

Some school systems employ "visiting teachers" who perform essentially the same duties as do school social workers. The teacher certification regulations of some states have been modified to permit nonteachers to become visiting teachers. In these circumstances, social workers often become visiting teachers.

Guidance Counselors

School guidance counselors provide two important kinds of service. They help students maximize their educational experience by assisting them in making decisions about course selection and advanced training, and they aid them in overcoming academic or social difficulties related to their school experience. School guidance counselors usually hold a master's degree in guidance and counseling from a graduate school of education. Many of them are particularly well qualified to work with students in a school setting because they were previously classroom teachers. Although guidance counselors have traditionally been employed in the high schools, there is a developing trend in some school systems to employ them in the elementary grades as well.

CHAPTER 8

Comprehensive Community Mental Health Centers

During the administration of the late President John F. Kennedy, Congress enacted comprehensive and far-reaching legislation which profoundly influenced the patterns of mental health service delivery throughout the country. Careful study by a task force showed that the mental health services available in the country were generally inadequate to meet the mental health needs of the people and that professional personnel were inefficiently distributed to meet the needs as the task force saw them. The coordination of existing services, from the consumer's viewpoint, was also seriously inadequate. Because of these conditions large numbers of citizens who sought mental health care ultimately became long-term patients in mental institutions with little hope of returning to productive and satisfying lives within their communities. If comprehensive and coordinated services were made available in all communities, many of these "custodial cases" might come to be treated early and close to home, thus precluding the necessity of later long-term institutionalization.

The result of these findings was legislation that provided for the formation and funding of comprehensive community mental health centers, envisioned as organizations that would coordinate the delivery of mental health services to the people of fixed geographic areas. The legislation provided that, if one or more essential mental health services were not available in an area, they be made accessible and integrated into the services already existing in the area. Thus, in regions with an abundance of services, the center might serve primarily as a coordinating agency. In areas with limited services the federal government would help to provide staffing and even buildings to make them available. There are hundreds of such centers in the United States today.

Community mental health centers are intended to provide a comprehensive and coordinated program of mental health services to the areas they serve. They are supposed to be close to where their clients live and to benefit local communities. The centers' services may occupy space attached to a hospital, or they may occupy a separate facility altogether. Whether the services are offered at one location or in a number of different ones, they should comprise a unified program permitting the patient to obtain continuity of timely and adequate mental health care. The mode of operation of these centers varies widely, with each reflecting the needs and resources of its own community.

Essential Services

The purpose of a community mental health center is to furnish a varied range of accessible and coordinated services designed both to prevent the occurrence of mental disorders and to treat existing ones. Most community mental health centers are funded by matching programs of the federal government (through the National Institute of Mental Health) and the local government. The majority of centers receive a large portion of their support from the federal government. In order to qualify for federal funds, a center must provide at least five essential services:

1. *Inpatient care,* offering treatment to patients who need residential care or hospitalization on a twenty-four hour per day basis.
2. *Outpatient care,* offering patients individual, group, or family therapy while permitting them to live at home and go about their daily lives.
3. *Partial hospitalization,* offering either day care for patients able to return to their homes in the evening or night care for patients able to work but in need of further care and who are usually without suitable home arrangements. It may include both day and night care and/or weekend care.
4. *Emergency care,* offering emergency mental health services at any hour at one or more of the above facilities.
5. *Consultation and education services,* offering assistance to local professional persons and agencies.

A community mental health center may offer more than the five essential services mentioned above. Additional services not required for federal support offer a more comprehensive program than the minimum stipulated services. Some additional services are:

1. *Diagnostic services,* including diagnostic evaluations and recommendations for appropriate treatment.
2. *Rehabilitative services,* including both social and vocational rehabilitation such as vocational testing, counseling, or job placement.
3. *Precare and aftercare,* providing screening of patients prior to hospital admission, home visits before and after hospitalization, follow-up services for clients of outpatient clinics, and partial hospitalization programs in foster or nursing homes or in halfway houses.
4. *Training programs,* offering training for all types of mental health workers who serve the center's patients or clients.
5. *Research and evaluation,* for evaluating the effectiveness of the center's programs and analyzing the needs of the area it serves. Mental health centers can also sponsor and conduct nonevaluative research projects such as demonstration projects or population surveys.
6. *Special services,* offering mental health care to a group of people with some particular mental health need in common. Examples of such special services might be drug-abuse programs, suicide prevention programs, and juvenile delinquency prevention programs. (The realities of today's world find many mental health centers involved with this kind of special service program.)

Making all of these services available locally and in a coordinated network represents the most advanced thinking. The coordination of these types of services enables the patient to move easily from one kind of treatment to another as his needs dictate. Moreover, the treatment can be carried out at any time that it is appropriate.

To help assure continuity of care, most mental health centers have a central record-keeping system which makes the patient's records readily available to authorized personnel of the various services of the center or to other associated agencies. These records, of course, are used only with the patient's permission.

The Catchment Area

Comprehensive community mental health centers must be available to all persons in the geographic area served by the center (the catchment area), without regard to age, race, creed, national origin, or ability to pay. A catchment area is defined by the federal government as an area of not less than 75,000 nor more than 200,000 persons. In an urban area, a center may serve an inner city neighborhood of up to 200,000 people. In rural regions, whole counties in one or adjacent states may join together to form a mental health center.

Inpatient Service

The inpatient service of the modern community mental health center is an essential link in the community mental health service system, since it insures continuity and variety of mental health care. Statistics show that 80 to 90 percent of all patients who receive intensive care in a local inpatient service show improvement within two to six weeks. These patients may then be transferred to another service in the community program for continuing treatment, for example, partial hospitalization or outpatient care. If the patient requires a longer period of hospitalization or if the demand for places in the hospital is acute, he may be transferred to a nursing home, a state mental hospital, or another residential treatment facility. In any case, however, the mental health center seeks to insure that the care he receives is both continuous and coordinated.

Inasmuch as hospitalization usually has a disruptive effect on people's lives, the inpatient unit is usually very careful in screening and evaluating a person's situation *before* admitting him to a residential treatment facility. There are, however, many different situations that might call for a person to be hospitalized. Certain individuals may require full-time hospitalization at the onset of their mental disorder or at some particularly stressful point during outpatient treatment. An individual requiring inpatient treatment may be referred to the service through the emergency unit of the center or by his physician, clergyman, community agency, or mental health therapist. By whatever route he is admitted, treatment will be aimed toward moving him into another service of the center as soon as he is enough improved to take the next step.

The inpatient service of the center is often a psychiatric unit of a general hospital affiliated with the community mental health program. Being cared for in a local and familiar hospital with family, friends, and family physician nearby for consultation can contribute significantly to speeding the patient's recovery.

The treatments most commonly employed in modern inpatient units are the various forms of psychotherapy and the somatic therapies, of which drug therapy is the most commonly used (see chapter 4). The physical needs of the patient are also given close attention in inpatient units. As a result of this attention, the staff sometimes detects neurological, metabolic, or other disorders which can cause and/or complicate mental disorders (see chapter 3). Medical facilities are almost always available to psychiatric patients either in the center where they are inpatients or through arrangements with a better-equipped hospital.

Outpatient Service

Many of the people who suffer from mental problems are able to go about their daily work and family lives while receiving care on an outpatient basis (see chapter 6). With new drugs and new treatment techniques literally thousands of people have been able to receive timely treatment in the hundreds of clinics that have been established across the country; and many of these clinics have become associated with community mental health centers, further expanding their potential for serving their communities. Available data indicate that, in 1966, for example, approximately one million Americans from all walks of life turned to more than two thousand mental health clinics for help. Among them were adults, children, and adolescents for whom the timely care received from a community outpatient service may have helped prevent a more prolonged and painful problem.

The outpatient service offers several unique benefits to the community. First, like the entire community mental health center program, outpatient services can easily be made accessible to everyone who lives within the center's catchment area. Second, the center's outpatient service is designed to carry out an active and flexible treatment program. Thus its various teams work with the assurance that back-up services are available through their own organization if their patients need them. The actual form of the outpatient service varies from center to center. In many areas an established clinic has become affiliated with a community hospital to form the outpatient facility. Sometimes the outpatient program has been established as a new service of a central facility that includes all the mental health services essential to providing continuity of patient care. In other areas the outpatient department of a general hospital operates the psychiatric service as part of a mental health center program. Whatever the arrangements, the outpatient service is an important link in the center's chain of services.

Partial Hospitalization

Partial hospitalization is designed for patients with mental or emotional disorders who spend only part of the day in a residential program. Partial hospital care can be an adaptable and flexible mode of treatment and it can differ from full hospitalization in several respects other than the duration of the hospital stay. It provides intensive mental health treatment while permitting the patient to continue his occupation or other activities. In this way it permits the patient to solve his emotional problem without creating additional problems that might arise if his whole life were disrupted by a period of isolated residential treatment.

Personnel in partial hospitalization programs usually include the same staff as in full hospitalization. Partial hospital care may be provided in any one of the facilities connected with the mental health center's program. In some centers, day or night care or both are provided at the local hospital, whereas in others partial hospitalization shares the building that houses the outpatient service. In still others, all services, including partial hospitalization, are located in one building.

Emergency Services

The emergency room of the general hospital is often the first place various mental problems are brought to the attention of the physician, nurse, and other health workers. It is becoming increasingly common for general hospitals to provide initial diagnosis of and treatment for these problems. Some general hospitals employ a psychiatrist, psychologist, and social worker as regular members of the emergency-room team. In addition, these professionals provide mental health consultation to other departments of the hospital.

The mental health emergency has been rather narrowly limited in concept to persons who behave in a way that seems to be dangerous to themselves or to others. It has traditionally been the function of families, clergymen, and the police to assist people experiencing such a problem. But modern thinking takes a broader point of view. Today it is known that mental health emergencies are not limited to persons who might possibly be dangerous; the troubled behavior of those who are given immediate professional attention often improves dramatically with timely treatment.

A large majority of people with mental disorders can respond to help and can recover. Just as immediate treatment for pneumonia, heart attacks, or other physical illnesses increases the likelihood of a favorable outcome, so does immediate treatment for mental problems increase the probability for success.

Who can benefit from mental health emergency services? Most professionals would agree that those conditions characterized by serious depression constitute a very high percentage of mental health emergencies. People in such condition are particularly in need of help because of the close link between serious depression and attempts at suicide. In many communities endeavors are made to prevent suicide by means of telephone answering services that operate twenty-four hours a day. One of the best known of these is the Suicide Prevention Center in Los Angeles which has been operating since 1958.

Another frequent form of mental health emergency involves people who experience some kind of "anxiety attack," usually expressed with panic, confusion, or bizarre behavior. These people may be neither suicidal nor threatening to others but are experiencing intense discomfort. They sometimes go of their own accord to a mental health facility to seek relief from their agitation and distress. In other cases a relative or friend who recognizes the need for help may escort the distressed person to the treatment facility.

Drunkenness is another major cause of mental health emergencies. For instance, a person who already suffers from some form of mental or emotional disturbance with which he can cope while sober may become panic-stricken under the influence of alcohol and become aggressive or behave unacceptably in some other way. Another mental health emergency associated with the overuse of alcohol is delirium tremens ("D.T.'s"). This condition is well known in hospitals, many of which classify it as a psychiatric disorder. The condition itself may be regarded more appropriately as a medical disorder since the person in delirium tremens may die if he does not receive prompt and specialized medical care. After the patient has been detoxified, however, he should receive a psychiatric examination and counseling to determine whether he will accept professional help in overcoming his excessive drinking.

It is common knowledge that bizarre and/or deviant behavior is manifested in persons under the effects of drugs or toxic elements that affect the central nervous system. Amphetamines, barbiturates, and LSD are common examples. As in the case of conditions caused by alcohol ingestion, these manifestations warrant prompt medical intervention and further psychiatric or neurological evaluation and management.

Prompt attention is also necessary when a person shows a convulsive disorder, regardless of etiology. Epilepsy and its severe manifestation, *status epilepticus* (a repeated and continuous convulsive episode which may have a lethal outcome), although a neurological disorder, are often regarded as mental health emergencies. They can be handled properly in a hospital facility or a mental health center.

Aggressive mentally disturbed people are relatively rare, yet it is in the interest of both the person and his community that there be provision for bringing seriously aggressive people to a mental health treatment facility immediately and in a humane way. Although treatment is often made easier when the patient is admitted voluntarily, the inpatient service of a center is prepared to receive persons who are committed by the courts.

Most emergency programs include a twenty-four-hour walk-in service, a twenty-four-hour telephone service, a service for suicide prevention, and in some cases even a home visiting service. The twenty-four-hour walk-in service essentially means that one can see a mental health professional at any time of the day or night without waiting any longer than his turn in the reception room. The twenty-four-hour telephone service provides round-the-clock consultation (anonymous if the caller wishes) with a mental health professional.

Consultation and Education

Consultation and education are an integral part of virtually every community mental health center's program. Their purpose is to extend the professional expertise of the center's staff to workers in other human services who have to deal with mental problems in the course of their daily activities—for example, policemen, judges, teachers, welfare workers, and clergymen. With such training they should be able to spot mental disorders early and see that they are treated in a timely and adequate way.

Gerald Caplan uses the term *consultation* "to denote a process of interaction between two professional persons—the consultant who is a specialist and the consultee who invokes the consultant's help in regard to a current work problem with which he is having some difficulty and which he has decided is within the other area of specialized competence. The work problem involves the management or treatment of one or more clients of the consultee, or the planning or implementation of a program to cater to such clients."[1] Technically there are many different types of mental health consultation, each of which can be characterized by its stated purpose, the setting in which it is offered, or the person or persons at whom it is directed.

Mental health education is a process by which factual information about some aspect of mental health is disseminated. A mental health center might, for example, offer specialized seminars in new approaches to psychotherapy for mental health professionals as well as courses for

1. Gerald Caplan, *The Theory and Practice of Mental Health Consultation* (New York: Basic Books, 1970), p. 19.

police officers on how to recognize mental problems. Virtually any topic related to the psychological well-being of the citizens of a community could be the subject of a mental health education program.[2]

What to Expect from Community Mental Health Centers

The official publication that spells out current operating procedures for mental health centers supported by federal funds is *Community Mental Health Center Program Operating Handbook* (MH-30102 11-70). This handbook is in looseleaf form and is being continuously updated.[3]

According to federal guidelines, a community mental health center should offer the following:

1. It should be a complete and readily available source of information about mental health services, facilities, practitioners, and programs within the community.
2. It should provide at least the five essential services described previously. The levels of the services should reflect the needs of the community as determined by its citizens.
3. Services provided by the center should be easy to find and use.
4. The center should make its services available in a prompt, efficient, and professional manner to everyone in the community regardless of age, sex, race, national origin, religion, or ability to pay.
5. The staff of the center as well as the people who govern its affairs should be representative of the people they serve. This is particularly applicable to language and cultural or ethnic background.
6. The center should be active and innovative in dealing with the mental health needs of its community.
7. It should spend a portion of its efforts and resources on the evaluation of its programs and activities.

2. B. W. MacLennan, R. D. Quinn, and D. Schroeder, *The Scope of Community Mental Health Consultation and Education*, National Institute of Mental Health, Public Health Service Publication No. 2169 (1971), U.S. Printing Office, 25 cents.

3. Copies of the handbook are available from the Handbook Coordination Officer, Management Policy Branch, OAM, National Institute of Mental Health, 5600 Fishers Lane, Rockville, Maryland 20852.

CHAPTER 9

Mental Health Services for Special Populations

Children

The development of services to meet the mental problems of children—as developing individuals—has been quite spotty when compared with the growth of similar services for the rest of the population. In addition to having some unique physical and mental needs, children as minors are subject to special conditions that have had important effects on the way mental health services have developed to meet their particular needs.

Historically, mental health services for children have not broadened in a comprehensive and coordinated manner. Where these services have developed, they have usually come about as adjuncts of other services such as schools and juvenile courts. Moreover, a young person in need of mental health services may have a double disadvantage in that he may be deemed unable to manage his own affairs both because of his mental status and because of his age. That is, he may be unable to represent his own interests because he is legally alleged to be doubly "incompetent." There are, however, some mental health services available to young people at various times as they grow and mature.

Medical Care for Infants

Parents of infants should make sure that their children have timely, regular, and continuing medical care to prevent a series of conditions that may be related to later mental problems or mental retardation. In addition to providing the appropriate immunizations (vaccines), the staff of the well-baby clinic (or a private physician or pediatrician) can spot the remedy conditions that, if untreated, can have lasting effects on the child and, indirectly, on his family. Phenylketonuria (PKU), a rare genetic anomaly, is a good example of such a condition. Untreated, PKU can result in mental retardation. But if the condition is recognized early (with a simple test) and if the child's diet is altered, later retardation can be prevented. Birth defects affecting hearing, sight, speech, posture, and coordinated movement can also contribute to the later development of mental disorders if they are left untreated. These conditions (e.g., cleft palates, harelips, crossed eyes) can be corrected most easily when they are recognized early and remedied promptly.

Care During Preschool Years

The preschool years offer parents a good opportunity both to prevent the later occurrence of mental problems and to minimize the effects of problems that do occur by seeking timely mental health services for their children.

There are a number of excellent books about child and baby growth and care available commercially or through government agencies (see chapter 10). These books provide the parents with a frame of reference for making preliminary judgments about behaviors that may indicate the beginning of a mental disorder. Just as important, they describe childhood behaviors that are perfectly normal.

In general, parents should be sensitive to either great changes in growth, or arrested growth, and certain sudden behavior changes that may signal the beginning of a mental problem. Self-destructive behavior, frequent temper tantrums, seriously withdrawn behavior, unusual fears, or difficulties with gait, muscle tone, coordination, or balance are examples of behaviors that may indicate the beginning of a mental or neurological disorder.

The physical environment in which a child lives can contribute to the development of mental disorders or mental retardation problems. For example, children who have chewed on objects coated with certain lead-based paints are sometimes known to suffer permanent, irreversible brain damage with associated mental retardation. Traumatic head injuries cause a number of children to be institutionalized every year because of associated behavior changes and/or retardation.

Finally, attention should be paid to the child's social environment.

Parents can do a lot to prevent mental problems by preparing their children for the potentially traumatic events that may occur in the life of almost every child. Two examples of such events are moving to another home and routine surgery requiring hospitalization. Hospitalization and surgery, even if they are medically minor, can be extremely stressful for some young children. (Examples of such minor operations include tonsillectomies, circumcision, and tooth extractions.) In order to minimize this stress and to prevent later emotional complications from developing, many hospitals have made arrangements for parents to "live in" with their children. Surgeons, anesthetists, and nurses are becoming increasingly aware of the psychological impact of even minor surgery and hospitalization on their young patients, and they are taking constructive steps to minimize the probability that psychological complications will arise from them.

Mental Health Service Settings for Children

Many mental health service organizations specialize in the diagnosis and treatment of the mental problems of young people. Child guidance centers and children's units of general and mental hospitals are examples. In some areas there are multiservice centers which offer a comprehensive range of services for children with serious emotional or neurological disorders. These centers are often funded directly by the city or the state. In the private sector are mental health professionals, such as psychiatrists, psychologists, and social workers, who specialize in the treatment of children. These professionals function as part of a team in the facilities just mentioned and sometimes in juvenile courts.

Juvenile courts. Juvenile courts are legal courts which make and execute decisions about children who have come to the attention of law enforcement agencies. It is important to note that a young person can come to the notice of the juvenile court either because some aspect of his behavior is unacceptable, or because he is a victim of a situation beyond his control (like neglect, abandonment, or abuse). The juvenile court, therefore, functions as a legal forum, a social agency, and a community referral resource all at once.

Some juvenile courts provide mental health evaluations as an "in-house" function while others can make them available on a contractual basis with agencies or by subsidizing the services of private practitioners. The probation staff of the court often monitor the mental health services provided by the court.

Battered and abused children. Many children come to the attention of the juvenile courts because they have been involved in brutal situations over which they had no control. Cases of child abuse and battered children are increasing to the point that in some cities there are special treatment units for these children (usually staffed by pediatricians, nurses, and social workers). Technically, an abused child is one who has been subjected to psychological abuse and/or neglect of a serious proportion. A battered child is one who has, in addition, suffered serious physical abuse from severe bruises to skull fractures, broken bones, and internal injuries resulting from heavy blows. When these children come to the attention of the juvenile courts, they are often placed in foster homes after receiving the necessary medical treatment.

Unfortunately, the majority of cases of child abuse never come to the notice of the courts because they are not reported. One reason is that in many areas the person who reports them (usually a physician who is called to treat the child's injuries) is vulnerable to legal retribution by the parents of the child. Some states, however, have recently taken steps to grant legal immunity to physicians who report instances of child battering to the authorities.

Adult Offenders: Services Through the Courts

The judicial systems of several states provide special mental health services to the courts, consisting mostly in mental health evaluations of accused offenders. These evaluations are made for the use of the court to give the judge information that may be relevant to the hearing and disposition of the accused offender's case. In this respect, the mental health services of the courts differ from those provided by the mental health service facilities discussed previously. That is, the evaluation services provided by the court are primarily for its use, although both prosecution and defense representatives may have access to the results. The evaluations may be carried out by the professional staff of the court clinic or on a contractual basis by a private practitioner (usually a psychiatrist).

If the defense attorney wishes to have an independent evaluation made of his client in order to serve the interest of his client, he may arrange for it by contracting a private practitioner for that purpose. In this case, the defendant or his attorney should arrange for the independent evaluation early in the pretrial process.

Mental health evaluations for adults involved in court proceedings may be divided into three phases: pretrial, trial, and presentence.

Pretrial phase. One of the main uses of mental health evaluations in the pretrial phase of a court proceeding is to determine the accused offender's competency to stand trial. This involves a determination of whether the offender knows the nature of the crime of which he is accused and whether he is able to assist in his own defense. Mental health evaluations may also be used to assist the court in an assessment of the behavior and overall personality of the defendant to determine whether further legal proceedings will be entertained by the court.

Trial phase. In some states a defendant may introduce expert testimony (usually by a psychiatrist) that relates to his mental status at the time of the crime. Such a defense strategy might be intended to convince the jury that the defendant's mental status was impaired at the time of the crime and, therefore, premeditation or the intent to commit the crime was absent or nonexistent.

Presentence phase. Once the legal issues of guilt or innocence have been resolved and the defendant has been found guilty of committing the crime, the court may require a psychiatric, psychological, and/or social work evaluation before sentencing. The results of these assessments, conveyed to the court in the form of a written document known as a presentence report, give the judge a better picture of the convicted defendant. The judge will carefully consider these findings, but it is his total responsibility to determine the final disposition of the case and the place where the sentence will be carried out (prison, mental hospital, or probation).

In probate courts, similar evaluation services may be provided to help the judge in the resolution of cases of child custody or adoption. There are several other kinds of legal proceedings where the psychiatrist, the psychologist, or the social worker might be called upon to render expert testimony. Some examples are cases involving workmen's compensation claims, civil suits, and cases involving alcohol or drug addiction.

Treatment Facilities in Courts and Correctional Institutions

Juvenile courts sometimes provide individual and/or group psychotherapy for parolees and for those in various detention facilities. They also frequently provide mental health services and consultation through detention homes, special camps, and vocational rehabilitation settings. These correctional facilities usually have access to a wide range of mental health services including neurological services.

Some prisons have hospitals with a mental health unit. Many prisons can choose from a wide range of mental health services for inmates, whereas others have troubleshooting clinics which function to identify specific problem areas within the institution and to bring in outside consultation to solve these problems where appropriate. Some progressive penal systems offer mental health services to the spouses and families of convicted offenders (like consultation, education, and family and group therapy).

Industry

Many industries provide both direct and indirect mental health services for employees and their families. Direct services include counseling concerning issues of work performance and conditions, promotions, retirement, and domestic relations. Individual psychotherapy is also available to employees of some organizations either by the professional staff of the company or subsidized by a health insurance plan. The "group therapy" offered by many companies to its management is really not psychotherapy in the usual sense but, rather, is designed to identify and remedy communication difficulties that may exist between people in the organization. Many companies also sponsor (or contribute to) rehabilitation programs for the benefit of employees with problems related to alcohol and/or drug use. Referral to community diagnostic and treatment facilities, as well as assistance in making arrangements with them, are also important direct mental health services offered to employees by many industrial and commercial companies.

Many organizations offer a broad range of direct services aimed at preventing mental disorders. The screening of personnel for positions to which they are best suited and the screening of employees to detect possible alcohol and drug use (often by urine and saliva tests) are examples of this kind of service. The development of day-care centers for the children of employees is a developing trend in industry that should have an important influence upon the future mental health of both employees and their families.

Mental health education, consultation, and seminars for executives, middle management, industrial physicians and nurses, and administrative personnel are examples of indirect mental health services provided by industrial or commercial organizations. Epidemiological studies, which seek to identify the specific conditions associated with mental disorders or physical injuries, are one of the most important indirect services provided to employees by industrial and commercial organizations. The findings of these studies are used not only to prevent these occurrences but also to plan facilities for the rehabilitation of those employees who have been affected by various industrial accidents, and mental problems, including alcoholism and drug abuse.

Minority Groups

"Minority group" is a loose phrase that could mean different things to different people. The term sometimes creates confusion because of the multiple implications and applications associated with it. It can refer, for example, to ethnic or racial background, cultural background, socioeconomic status, religious belief, or area of residence. It is usually used in reference to poverty or racial origin. The term as used here refers to certain groups of people with some specific mental problem in common, who have a particular need for a specific kind of mental health service, and who are considered to be socioeconomically disadvantaged.

A member of a minority group may find that his race, language, socioeconomic status, or area of residence is related to his inability to get the service he needs. For example, a poor black person and a poor white person from a rural area might have in common a shared inability to get timely and adequate mental health services near their homes. A black person and a Spanish-speaking person living in city ghettos might share the same unfortunate communality. Sometimes, then, a person who is a member of a minority group might make good use of mental health services but for the fact that his access to those services is limited. Language or cultural differences between the care givers and those seeking mental health services could also be limiting factors to be reckoned with either because the professional persons and the potential clients are unable to communicate verbally, or because they do not attach the same relevance to the definition and solution of mental problems and other human dilemmas. Unfortunately, mistrust between care givers and potential clients grows very rapidly in such a climate.

Community workers who may have occasion to assist a minority group or a non-English-speaking person to get appropriate mental health services should consider the following courses of action:

1. Inquiries can be made in the neighborhood about what mental health services are available.
2. If there is a problem communicating in English, it is worth finding out if someone connected with the local mental health facilities speaks the client's language. Possibly, some local mental health facilities have either an employee or a consultant who does.
3. If there is no one available who can verbally communicate with the individual seeking mental health services, translation services might be available through the church, the language department of the local high school, or through community self-help groups. There is an important trend developing today toward the formation of community-based self-help groups formed around some cultural, geographic, or linguistic communality shared by community members.
4. If some mental health services are available, particularly through a community mental health center, but access to those services is limited for reasons of language, it is in the interest of the community to provide the necessary interpretation services on a continuing basis.
5. Any mental health program receiving federal funds is required to make its services available to all people regardless of race, ethnic background, religion, or sex; more than that, however, the composition of the staffs of these organizations is supposed to reflect the population it serves. If difficulty in receiving mental health services

is related to either of these factors, one should request a review and improvement of the situation from *both* the care-giving agency *and* the federal agency providing the funds. To find out if a mental health service facility is receiving federal funds, a written inquiry should be addressed to the National Clearinghouse for Mental Health Information (see chapter 10). If a citizen feels that he is being discriminated against by virtue of receiving inadequate or inappropriate mental health services and if the agency he is dealing with is the recipient of government funds, he may also seek satisfaction through the state human rights commission, by petitioning elected officials, or by engaging legal counsel.

6. Finally, if a client of a mental health service facility suspects that there is a significant language or value gap between himself and the staff members, extra care should be taken in negotiating a therapeutic contract.

CHAPTER 10

Some Sources of Mental Health Information

There must be thousands of groups, organizations, and associations involved in one way or another in the field of mental health. Just about every month a new research finding, a new technique, a new medication, or a new law appears to change "what is happening" in this already complex field. As a result, no single book could be a complete or current directory of mental health information or services; yet one must have a starting point, or key, that will facilitate purposeful entry into the diffuse mental health information network. This chapter will present a few such keys.

Anyone in need of detailed and current information about something related to mental health should be able to obtain it quickly by addressing an inquiry to the appropriate sources listed below. Although these represent only a small fraction of the possible sources of mental health information that exist in the United States, they have been selected because each is a respected source of current information and because each will, if necessary, lead to other sources of information which cannot be listed in a book of this length.

Information Sources at the National Level

National Professional Associations

A consumer of mental health services can make use of national professional associations in a number of ways:

1. As a source of general mental health information such as books, pamphlets, and other printed materials.

2. As a source of specific answers to specific questions.
3. As a source of information about individual professional persons contained in membership lists and directories. These directories frequently contain a summary of the training and experience of each professional member.
4. As a way to locate state and local chapters of the association.
5. As a sensitive place to address complaints about specific activities of individual professional persons. (Most professional associations have standing committees on ethics and professional practice.)

The names and addresses of selected national professional associations are:

American Psychiatric Association (APA)
1700 Eighteenth Street, NW
Washington, D.C. 20009

American Psychological Association (APA)
1200 Seventeenth Street, NW
Washington, D.C. 20036

National Association of Social Workers (NASW)
600 Southern Building
Fifteenth and H Streets, NW
Washington, D.C. 20005

American Board of Psychiatry and Neurology (ABPN)
P.O. Box 1157
Rochester, Minnesota 55902

American Academy of Neurology (AAN)
4005 W. Sixty-Fifth Street
Minneapolis, Minnesota 55435

American Board of Professional Psychology, Inc. (ABPP)
Address of current Executive Secretary available through American Psychological Association (above).

American Psychoanalytic Association (APA)
1 East Fifty-Seventh Street
New York, New York 10022

Association for the Advancement of Behavior Therapy (AABT)
415 East Fifty-Second Street
New York, New York 10022

Behavior Therapy and Research Society
c/o Eastern Pennsylvania Psychiatric Institute
Henry Avenue
Philadelphia, Pennsylvania 19129

American Group Psychotherapy Association (AGPA)
1790 Broadway
Room 702
New York, New York 10019

American Medical Association (AMA)
535 N. Dearborn Street
Chicago, Illinois 60610

National Medical Association (NMA)
1108 Church Street
Norfolk, Virginia 23510

American Academy of General Practice (AAGP)
Special Committee on Mental Health
Volker Boulevard at Brookside
Kansas City, Missouri 64112

American Nurses Association (ANA)
2420 Pershing Road
Kansas City, Missouri 64108

National Education Association (NEA)
1201 Sixteenth Street, NW
Washington, D.C. 20036

American Bar Association (ABA)
1155 E. Sixtieth Street
Chicago, Illinois 60637

Units of the Federal Government

The federal government is the single most important force in the field of mental health today. Through its several offices, bureaus, and institutes, it supports the delivery of mental health services, sponsors vast dollar amounts for research, supports individuals and institutions engaged in professional training programs, and contributes heavily to the actual building of mental health facilities. It also collects an enormous amount of mental health information that it will make available (either free or at minimal cost) to those who request it.

U. S. Department of Health, Education, and Welfare (HEW). The Department of Health, Education, and Welfare is the cabinet level of the government that bears the major direct responsibility for mental health matters. HEW is composed of a vast and complex network of institutes, divisions, and offices, many of which are involved with mental health matters in one way or another. There is, however, one important office that has as its primary purpose making all kinds of mental health information available to citizens. Consequently, one of the best keys to HEW is:

National Clearinghouse for Mental Health Information
National Institute of Mental Health
Parklawn Building
5600 Fishers Lane
Rockville, Maryland 20852

Another repository of information within HEW is the U.S. Office of Education. This office provides information about mental health activities and programs in the schools. Inquiries may be addressed to:

U.S. Office of Education
Federal Office Building 6
400 Maryland Avenue, SW
Washington, D.C. 20202

The Health Services and Mental Health Administration (HSMHA) is a very important part of HEW since it has direct control over large sums of money that are used directly to subsidize local mental health services, particularly community mental health centers. HSMHA would be an appropriate place to direct specific technical questions about the fiscal administration of community mental health centers. Of interest to this source, for example, are accurately documented accounts of improper or inadequate functioning concerning any of the facilities it supports. Inquiries may be addressed to:

Health Services and Mental Health Administration
Parklawn Building
5600 Fishers Lane
Rockville, Maryland 20852

U.S. Department of Housing and Urban Development (HUD). The U.S. Department of Housing and Urban Development is a cabinet-level department of the federal government that supports some activities related to mental health. One of the most widely known activities of this department is the Model Cities program. Inquiries may be addressed to:

U.S. Department of Housing and Urban Development
451 Seventh Street, NW
Washington, D. C. 20410

U.S. Department of Justice. The Justice Department is a cabinet-level department of the federal government that supports a good deal of activity related to certain legal aspects of mental health. The Law Enforcement Assistance Administration (LEAA) is a relatively new unit of the Justice Department that is engaged in a number of research projects, pilot projects, training programs, and direct services related to mental health. Inquiries may be addressed to:

Law Enforcement Assistance Administration
U. S. Department of Justice
633 Indiana Avenue, NE
Washington, D.C. 20530

U.S. Government Printing Office. The U.S. Government Printing Office has the responsibility each year of printing and distributing (either free or at minimal cost) tons of material, much of it involving mental health and special education. One of the most useful things this office does is to circulate periodic mailing lists which describe new publications dealing with particular topics, together with instructions on how to get them. Inquiries about available publications or about having one's name placed on a particular mailing list may be sent to:

Superintendent of Documents
U. S. Government Printing Office
Washington, D. C. 20402

U.S. Social Security Administration and Veterans Administration.
The Social Security Administration subsidizes certain mental health
services for eligible citizens. In addition to providing certain mental-
health-related services, the U.S. Veterans Administration actually offers mental health services directly to eligible veterans and other qualifying persons. These two governmental agencies, for all their differences,
share a common characteristic that is important both to citizens seeking information and to those presenting claims. Both of these large organizations are quite decentralized; that is, much of their activity takes
place in regional offices. The addresses of regional offices may be obtained at any local post office.

Congressmen and Senators

Congressmen and senators are local and state representatives in
Washington, and in certain circumstances they can be of great help to
consumers of mental health services. When they are called upon to
"play offense" they can help to expedite the development of new mental health programs and services that are supported in whole or in part
by federal funds. "On defense" they can help to insure the continued
existence of federally funded programs and services that are of value to
their constituents. Congressmen and senators welcome an opportunity
to assist constituents in procuring legitimately needed mental health services because it is their sworn responsibility to represent the legitimate
interests and sentiments of their constituents, and because satisfied
constituents tend to become supporters at election time. Consequently,
no one should be reluctant to ask his congressman and/or senator to
take a personal and active interest in speeding legitimate requests for
mental health services and programs through the ponderous federal
machinery.

National Mental Health Special-Interest Groups

There are several national organizations that are concerned with some
specific interest in a particular mental health matter. Most of these fur-

nish timely printed information, answers to specific questions, the services of a film library, and even an informed speaker for a church event or other gathering. Because these groups are active in promoting activities within their particular area of interest, they provide channels for constructive mental health volunteer activity through association with their local chapters. Some of these special-interest groups are:

National Association for Mental Health
10 Columbus Circle
New York, New York 10019

National Committee Against Mental Illness
1028 Connecticut Avenue
Washington, D. C. 20036

Council for Exceptional Children
c/o National Education Association
1201 Sixteenth Street, NW
Washington, D. C. 20036

National Association for Retarded Children
420 Lexington Avenue
New York, New York 10077

General Service Board of Alcoholics Anonymous (AA)
P. O. Box 459
Grand Central Station
New York, New York 10077

American Civil Liberties Union (ACLU)
156 Fifth Avenue
New York, New York 10010

Information Sources at the State Level

State Professional Associations

Most national professional associations have chapters or affiliated organizations which operate at the state level. These may be located by writing to the national organization's offices.

Units of State Government

In addition to providing citizens with information about matters related to mental health, various units of state government also support, maintain, and control the delivery of direct mental health services. These units of state government will usually be found in the capital city of the state.

State department of mental health (or mental hygiene). State departments of mental health usually have a public information officer who answers general inquiries addressed to the department. Besides furnishing information to interested citizens, these departments also operate a network of mental health service facilities including state mental hospitals, outpatient clinics, diagnostic centers, day-care centers, and so forth.

It is important to note that state departments of mental health can sometimes provide direct mental health services even though they do not actually operate the service-giving facility. Massachusetts, for example, has room in state mental hospitals for less than two hundred children at any particular time. Yet the department of mental health together with the department of education pay the bills for more than six hundred children in private mental hospitals, many of which are actually located in other states. Other departments of state government, like the department of welfare, can also pay for mental health treatment in private facilities under special circumstances. Such programs are not well publicized, and unless interested parents are persistent and resourceful, they may have difficulty obtaining specific information about them.

State department of education (or public instruction). State departments of education directly subsidize special education programs in several states and certify diagnosticians and special education teachers. In addition, they specify the regulations (eligibility requirements) under which the various special education programs operate.

State office of licensing and accreditation. The state offices of licensing and accreditation have the responsibility for issuing licenses and certificates to people who are qualified to practice the various professions that are officially regulated within the state. These offices can be sources of information about the license and certificate regulations as well as the status, relative to those regulations, of individual professional persons.

State Representatives and State Senators

Like their federal counterparts, state representatives and senators are local representatives in the state capital. They can be of assistance to concerned citizens either in the preservation of existing mental health services or in the development of legitimately needed new services and programs. They can also assist in rectifying documented instances of inadequate or improper mental health services that occur within their districts.

The Governor's Office

The governors of several states have established special suboffices within their executive offices to deal with certain matters of special interest within their respective states. Offices that might be helpful in providing information or assistance in finding services are the governor's office for consumer affairs, and the governor's office for drug abuse problems. (We wish to emphasize the function rather than the titles of these offices, as the exact titles vary from state to state.)

State Planning Commissions

One of the most important activities of the governor's office in every state is the state planning commission (or committee, or council, or other appropriate term). These organizations represent a point in the mental health service delivery chain where informed citizens can have a particularly strong impact. The commissions are composed of people appointed by the governor for the purpose of developing a statewide plan for coordinating existing services and programs and for developing priorities for adding new services in an orderly way to the network of services already available. Mental health is just one part of the state's comprehensive plan. (The state plan is a document that can be obtained by every citizen.)

One reason for state planning committees and state plans is that there is a new kind of relationship developing between state governments and the federal government, especially those units of the federal government which support or contribute to activities within the states. The result of all this is that the federal government has asked each state government, through its governor's office, to determine how it wants coordinated and comprehensive services to develop within its own territory. The planning committees appointed by the governor work this plan out and submit it to the federal government. The federal funding agencies then use the state plan as a working guideline for awarding a large percentage of the federal funds which go into that particular state. For example, if a request for a mental health program is submitted to a unit of the federal government and if that particular type of program has a low-priority ranking in the state's plan, that program, no matter how good and worthwhile it seems, will have a dismal chance of being funded.

Interested citizens might qualify by their area of residence, occupation, or ethnic background for membership on, or association with, one or several state planning agencies. They can inquire about these possibilities by writing to one of their state representatives or to the governor's office. Before taking that step, however, it would be a good idea to carefully research the membership requirements and the actual composition of the planning commissions of their state. If such a plan of action exceeds a person's ambitions or available time, he could still attend an occasional public hearing of the planning commissions. He could also request that such hearings be held in his community about issues of direct concern to that community.

Information Sources at the Local Level

Virtually every community in the United States contains at least one source of information about mental health services; and, a large proportion of these communities contains at least one source of mental health service. Some good starting points for obtaining information follow.

Community Mental Health Center

The first and most logical place to seek mental health information is a community mental health center. In fact, one of the primary reasons for the existence of these centers is to provide information and assistance to citizens about mental health matters. If the community mental health center does not provide adequate information (this would be very rare), interested citizens could help themselves and their neighbors by becoming actively involved in its operation as a volunteer, as a member of the board of directors, or in some other constructive capacity. If the community is not served by a community mental health center, interested citizens could take steps to start one (see chapter 11).

Local Agencies and Institutions

Local agencies and institutions are often good sources of mental health information. The following is a partial list of such public service organizations: general hospitals, particularly emergency and psychiatric services; mental hospitals; outpatient clinics; public schools; social agencies; courts, particularly juvenile and probate courts; state, county, and city police departments; Legal Aid Society and/or Public Defender's Office; the American Red Cross; the local public library; and the editor of the local newspaper.

Local Professional Persons

Individual professionals such as psychiatrists, psychologists, and social workers, are excellent sources of local mental health information because of their direct involvement in the field. Family physicians, lawyers, and clergymen are also valuable sources of information and advice about mental health matters. If they are unable, for ethical or practical reasons, to provide satisfactory answers, they will probably suggest some source where the information can be obtained.

Local Chapters of Mental Health Interest Groups

Many national mental health special-interest groups have active local chapters that supply mental health information. In addition to these associations, a number of locally based organizations such as parent-teacher organizations, chapters of Alcoholics Anonymous, and a multitude of self-help groups have information services. A list of these organizations can be obtained from the community relations office or the office of volunteer services of a mental hospital, general hospital, or other institution in the community.

Elected Local Officials

Local governments contribute to the financial support of mental health services delivered within their jurisdictions. The mayor, city manager, city council members, and county supervisors can help on the local level in the same ways that state and federal representatives can at their respective levels of government. Members of the county board of supervisors are sometimes overlooked by citizens as sources of assistance in mental health matters, probably because they are not as politically conspicuous as some other elected officials. County supervisors frequently exert a powerful influence on the delivery of local mental health services because community mental health centers, being regional rather than municipal agencies, are often under their direct fiscal control. Consequently, they are in a good position to rectify improper or inadequate services, or to help interested citizens become involved in the operation of the center if other channels for becoming involved are closed.

CHAPTER 11

Encouraging Citizen Participation in Mental Health Activities

Informed and effective citizens can promote mental health and help alleviate mental disorders by becoming directly involved in the planning and delivery of mental health services in their community. There is much important work to be done, many exciting discoveries waiting to be made, and a great deal of personal satisfaction to be gained by becoming personally involved in some aspect of the mental health field.

Many experts believe that an effective and efficient system of mental health services has to include both professional specialists and informed citizens. Professional specialists can determine the technicalities of how a particular mental health problem may be solved, but informed citizens and consumers of mental health services should determine what problems are to be worked on and in what order the work will proceed. This is where the citizen's contribution is important. After all, in addition to being directly affected by the quality and availability of mental health services, he is also paying the bills for these services with taxes, insurance premiums, and private dollars. Furthermore, there are probably as many different ways of becoming constructively involved in the mental health field as there are different people. An important contribution can usually be made by a person with sufficient interest, ability, and available time.

Participating as an Informed Citizen

Informed citizens can make a vital contribution to the delivery of mental health services by becoming actively involved in the influencing of political decisions. These decisions are made at various levels of the political system, and their effects, for good or for ill, are likely to be felt by large numbers of people.

State Comprehensive Health Plan

Every state has developed (or is developing) a comprehensive health plan as a guideline for the operation and development of a broad range of integrated human services. The committees or councils that formulate these plans and monitor their operation are especially important because they determine the priorities according to which mental health services (and others) will be developed and/or made available to the public. They are able to enforce conformity with these priorities because they have the ability to influence decisions about those projects and programs which will receive state and federal funds to support them, and those which will not. This, of course, is a highly political activity since the persons chosen to make these important decisions are usually appointed by the governor. (See "State Planning Commissions" in chapter 10.)

Unfortunately, the general public does not seem to be aware of the existence of these committees, nor does it know about what they are doing. It is possible that the people who have been chosen to make these decisions in some states have personal preferences or represent groups whose desires for mental health services are quite different from, or even prejudicial to, that of the majority of citizens. Even if one knows who these people are, it is still possible that they might not be constructively responsive to the majority's interests. There are, however, a number of steps that a citizen can take to minimize the probability that such an unhappy situation will materialize. First, he must educate himself about the committee and about the state plan. As a first step, he might write to his governor and ask for a copy of the state comprehensive health plan. He might also ask for a list of planning council members so that he can address inquiries to members from his area or to those who might represent a group of which he is also a member. Once he knows what the guidelines are and who is responsible for them, he will have taken the first step in becoming constructively involved in the decision-making process.

An interested citizen might, for example, take steps to become involved with one of the subcommittees or advisory groups of the council working on some aspect of mental health service that is of particular local interest. If some special interest of the community is not reflected in the existing plan, steps can be taken to remedy the situation by writing informed letters to various elected representatives, or by mobilizing a group of people with similar interests in order to bring about the desired change by applying political pressure or alerting public attention to the problem. Not infrequently, the citizen will end up appointed to the planning committee itself.

The State Department of Mental Health

Many state departments of mental health have attempted to make mental health services more responsive to the needs of citizens by decentralizing their operations. Decentralization usually involves dividing the state into several regions, each of which has its own administrative structure for delivering and coordinating the mental health services within its boundaries. The regions can be further subdivided into service-delivery areas. Where such a decentralized system is in operation, there should be an administrator (who is a state employee) available and responsible to every locality in the state.

Each region and area should also have a citizen advisory committee whose function is to convey the needs of the citizens living in a given area to the (decentralized) administrative staff of the department of mental health responsible for providing services to that area. If a state has a decentralized system of mental health service delivery, one can find out about becoming involved with the citizen council by addressing an inquiry to the local regional administrator or to the chairman of the council. The names and addresses of these people, together with information about the organization of the state's mental health service delivery system, may be obtained from the public information officer of the state department of mental health (see chapter 10).

Existing Community Mental Health Centers

Most community mental health centers receive a good deal of their financial support from the federal government, although some support comes from local units of government. (The proportions vary from center to center.) As a result, the governing bodies of these centers are supposed to be open, public, and representative of the people they serve. Any interested citizen is entitled to play a part in formulating the policies that guide the operation of his community mental health center. Just what part he will play depends on his interests, abilities, and available time. The main governing body of the mental health center is the board of directors. Any citizen should be eligible to be considered for a position as a board member. The board of directors frequently relies on a citizen advisory committee which is usually larger and more transient than the board itself. Citizens can inquire at the center about volunteering their services to the committee. They can also attend certain board and advisory committee meetings as observers.

If a citizen is satisfied with the way his community mental health center is operating and with its services, he should make his feelings known to the board of directors. They deserve informed support in order to make sure that a satisfactory level of mental health services will continue to be available to the community.

If, on the other hand, a citizen is dissatisfied with the adequacy or distribution of services within a community, he should make this known as well. If the complaint is not satisfactorily rectified by the board, he may still influence the operation of the center by presenting a documented case to elected representatives and to the officials who control the funds that support the center (see chapter 10).

Starting a New Community Mental Health Center

If a community does not have mental health center and a group of citizens would like to establish one, they can obtain a wealth of information from the National Institute of Mental Health (NIMH), which can supply detailed instructions and expert consultation as well as considerable financial support, even in the preliminary stages of starting a new center (see chapter 10). In fact, preliminary or initiation grants of up to $50,000 can be awarded by NIMH for this purpose.

It may be that a community has been deemed eligible for a center and that one is already in the planning stages. The National Institute of Mental Health will put interested citizens in touch with the people in the community who are doing the planning. Becoming involved early in the planning stage of a community mental health center is a very effective way to influence the subsequent delivery of services.

Mayor's Committees

The mayors of many communities convene special committees to investigate specific local problems. Many of these committees are involved with matters directly related to the mental health of the community or to the delivery of specific mental health services. Such committees might deal with drug abuse, alcoholism, police-community relations, halfway houses, mental health programs in the schools, or any of a number of other issues related to mental health.

Citizens can usually become involved with these committees or associated study groups simply by making their interest known. If a citizen has a special skill or talent, he will be doubly welcome on such a committee. An exserviceman, a nurse, or someone who can speak Spanish, for example, may find membership on one of these committees a constructive and rewarding way to promote the mental health of the community.

Church Groups

Churches often sponsor activities directly related to the promotion of mental well-being. Traditionally, church groups have had an important impact upon the delivery of mental health services within the community by organizing members to visit mental patients, prisoners, orphans, and residents of institutions for the mentally retarded. Not only has this attention had beneficial effects on the individuals visited, but these church groups have quietly altered the distribution of mental health services within many communities by persistently focusing attention on various groups of the "forgotten." In fact, some churches, like the Salvation Army, spend a good deal of their official energies on the rehabilitation of people who may well have serious mental problems.

More recently churches and church groups have become involved in activities designed to prevent or minimize the occurrence of mental disorders. They establish and sponsor "drop-in" counseling centers for young people and encourage members to provide foster homes for homeless children. Churches also support a wide variety of mental hospitals, social agencies, and institutions for the mentally retarded. Additional information about the mental health activities of church groups can be obtained by contacting one's clergyman.

Special-Interest Groups

It is quite possible that one or more national special-interest groups has an active local chapter in the community. One can find out about these groups by writing to the appropriate national headquarters (see chapter 10). There may also be local special-interest groups operating within the community. Information about these groups can be obtained by addressing an inquiry to the community relations officer of the local state mental hospital or the public information officer of the state department of mental health. If there is a community mental health center, that facility would be the most logical place to inquire initially.

Groups like the state mental health association or the state association for emotionally disturbed children usually provide a good deal of support for local mental health treatment facilities, in addition to carrying on a continuing educational program for their members. Such groups are always looking for new members, so an inquiry would be welcomed.

The United Fund

The United Fund supports a number of mental health services within each community and furnishes an exceptional vehicle for becoming constructively involved in a wide spectrum of mental health activities. Depending upon one's particular interests and abilities, the United Fund can provide opportunities for fund-raising, surveying existing mental health service facilities, planning for new programs, and many other important activities related to the mental health service system in the community. It can also help locate a mental health activity that both needs the citizen's assistance and meets his interest. Next to the community mental health center, the United Fund office is probably the best place to find out what is happening in mental health in the community.

Participating as a Volunteer

People with certain personalities work particularly well with others who are receiving mental health services. For such people, there is an almost limitless number of agencies and clients who are in need of their time and talents as volunteer workers. A few possibilities are discussed below.

Advocacy Service

In most communities there are organizations whose purpose is to insure that the rights of all citizens, including people with psychological problems, are preserved and respected. One such organization is the American Civil Liberties Union (ACLU). The ACLU provides a means for involvement in this vital enterprise. One need not be a lawyer to avail himself of this opportunity. Specific information about the ACLU, its activities, and its various local organizations may be obtained by writing directly to the national headquarters (see chapter 10).

Many communities have legal aid clinics which provide legal services for those who are unable to procure them for themselves. Many of the legal problems that the clinics handle are related in some way to mental health services. Examples might be commitment proceedings, issues related to competence to stand trial, and guardianship cases involving minors. The professional staffs of these organizations are qualified and dedicated attorneys, but the organizations still need a great deal of help in order to function at maximum efficiency. Consequently there may be opportunities to contribute to the activities of a legal aid clinic by volunteering as a receptionist, bookkeeper, typist, researcher, or general office helper.

Many community organizations like schools and government agencies have rediscovered the utility of an ombudsman, a kind of referee who resolves disputes that arise between people with conflicting interests. In addition to being skillful, impartial, and resourceful in the settlement of disputes, the person who occupies such a delicate position must have the confidence of both parties involved in the conflict, because under this system both must agree to abide by the decision of the ombudsman. If a school system, social agency, governmental department, or mental health service facility in his community is considering instituting such a system, and if he has the qualifications *and* the disposition, an interested citizen might volunteer his services as an ombudsman.

Service in Institutions and Clinics

Most mental health service facilities need many more volunteers than are actually available to them. Because of this situation, anyone interested is virtually assured of an opportunity to become involved in the activities of these organizations in a great variety of ways. Information about these possibilities may be gathered by contacting the coordinator of volunteer services at the local mental hospital, the local United Fund office, or the community mental health center. The possibilities for this kind of voluntary involvement are almost limitless, so only a few of them will be listed.

Some people may, for example, want to volunteer a few hours per week in the direct care of mental patients. In this capacity, one could assist the nurses and attendants of the hospital by escorting the patients from place to place, or by helping individual patients to write letters to their families or to complete schoolwork; or one might prefer to volunteer his aid to the social services department of the hospital by serving as a typist, receptionist, or general office worker. The occupational and recreational therapists may make use of a volunteer's services in helping a patient or two complete a project, or by making it known to their patients that he will be available at certain times to join in a basketball game or in a stroll on the hospital grounds. The possibility of sharing a hobby, like model-building, sewing, or photography, with the patients of an institution should not be overlooked. A valuable service can also be provided by driving people to and from various appointments or by volunteering to drive patients' families to and from the hospital for visits.

Finally, one might volunteer to help with activities away from the institution—for example, escorting a patient or two to a baseball game or on some other kind of outing. A volunteer can also provide respite from institutional life by having a patient come to his home for an occasional Sunday or holiday dinner. Of course, the staff of the institution will carefully screen the patients who are eligible for this privilege and will counsel the host in advance about the details of the visit.

CHAPTER 12

Conclusion

This book was written to provide some guidelines for obtaining and evaluating mental health services. Although it is addressed primarily to community workers with the responsibility of guiding people in need to and through the mental health service system, we hope that its ultimate beneficiaries will be the people who need mental health services and their families.

In the long run, providing conventional mental health services to individuals and their families can only be a partial solution to the national mental health problem, no matter how efficiently those services are provided. At the societal level many serious mental problems are associated with the tragic influences of war, poverty, racial prejudice, inadequate education, inhumane working conditions, unsatisfactory housing, malnutrition, environmental contamination, and the increasing mobility of our population. And, of course, these stressful events cannot be divorced from economic and political factors. So it seems to us that the time has come for both the providers and the consumers of mental health services to expand their horizons beyond the concepts of physical health, mental health, or even comprehensive health. We really need to begin dealing with the concept of human services which respects the integrity of the whole, complex human being by providing him with the various services he requires in a coordinated and integrated manner. There are, as a matter of fact, developments in various parts of the United States that seem to be leading in this direction. Three such developments will be mentioned here, and these have a very important element in common: the potential to make the providers of services more accountable to the consumers of those services.

When a plan of national health care becomes a reality, it will profoundly influence public human service facilities like state mental hospitals. In the past, the patients of these facilities had no choice about where they received mental health services either because they had no money or because they were hospitalized against their wills. A national health plan will give the clients of state mental hospitals a choice about where they receive mental health services because, to some extent at least, they will be able to pay for their treatment in either public or private facilities. It is hoped that this development will make both public and private facilities more efficient and effective treatment centers by introducing an element of healthy competition.

Second, involuntary commitment to mental hospitals is becoming less common and new laws are being enacted to protect the rights of patients of state mental hospitals. In Massachusetts, for example, a recently passed law permits involuntary commitment to state mental hospitals only in those cases where the patient is proved to be dangerous to himself or to others. Most important, however, is a provision of the Massachusetts statute mentioned earlier which requires state hospitals to review periodically each patient and to furnish him or his guardians with a written report outlining the treatment goals, a list of all treatments given and response to those treatments, a list of alternatives to hospitalization that have been explored, and, if further residential treatment is recommended, the reasons for that recommendation.

Finally, a few states are already reorganizing the framework within which the various human services are delivered. These reorganizations place several service departments, like public health, mental health, and welfare, under the direct control of a secretary of human services, who is responsible for coordinating the services provided by these departments and for allocating funds among them. This trend promises to introduce an element of constructive competition into the delivery of human services because, among other things, it obliges the individual departments to account for the elements of service they are delivering in more explicit and accountable ways. Massachusetts and Georgia are examples of states that have reorganized this way.

It appears that the developments just described have initiated a trend favoring the emergence of more general, coordinated services, and the trend toward greater and greater specialization—marked by professional isolation and consumer ignorance—is beginning to slow down. In order for these two opposing trends to come to an equilibrium favorable to both providers and consumers of mental health services, three conditions are essential:

1. Consumers of all kinds of human services (mental health services included) will have to become educated and discriminating users of the services already available to them.
2. Care givers and professional persons will have to be reeducated so that they will cooperate rather than compete with one another.
3. A new kind of alliance will have to evolve between providers and consumers of human services which favors cooperation and collaboration over fragmented, superspecialization.

If these conditions can be realized we will have made a quantum leap toward the realization of human potential and the alleviation of human misery.

Index

Index

Council for Exceptional Children, 115
Council on Social Work Education, 18
Courts: and involuntary commitment, 46, 55, 56, 57, 59; juvenile, 102–03, 105; services through, 69, 81, 103–05

Developmental disabilities: special classes for, 83–84
Diagnosis, 6–7, 22–24; interviews as part of, 24–25; examinations as part of, 25–34; sociocultural, 35–36; team approach to, 36–37; in mental hospitals, 61–62, 63; in mental health clinics, 78–79
Diagnostic labels, 7–8
Drug treatment. *See* Chemotherapy

Echoencephalography, 30
Educational achievement tests, 34
Electroconvulsive therapy (ECT), 47, 49
Electroencephalogram (EEG), 28–29, 63
Emergencies: locating help in, 20–21; walk-in clinics, 20, 43, 73–74, 98; hot lines, 20, 74, 98
Emergency services: in mental hospitals, 60; in mental health clinics, 73–74; in classrooms, 88; in community mental health centers, 91, 95–98; in general hospitals, 95–96
Examinations. *See* Medical specialty examinations

Family therapy, 44–45
Fees. *See* Cost of services; Sliding-fee schedules
Federal government: as information source, 109–15
Freud, Anna, 41
Freud, Sigmund, 40, 41

Group psychotherapy, 43–44
Guidance counselors, 89

Halfway houses, 60
Health Services and Mental Health Administration, 112–13
Hot lines, 20, 74, 98

Industry: psychiatry in, 12; mental health services in, 71, 105–06
Infants: medical care for, 100–01
Information release, 36
Information sources. *See* Mental health information sources
Inpatient treatment facilities, 91, 93–94. *See also* Mental hospitals
Insulin coma treatment, 50
Intelligence quotient (I.Q.), 33
Intelligence tests, 32–34
Interview. *See* Mental health interview

Juvenile courts, 102–03, 105

Law Enforcement Assistance Administration, 113
Licenses. *See* Certification and licensing
Lobotomy, 50–51
Local government: as information source, 120

Medical model, 40
Medical specialty examinations, 25; in mental hospital procedures, 63. *See also* Neurological examinations; Psychological tests
Mental health: concept of, 3–5, 6
Mental health activities: participation in, 121
—as informed citizen: state comprehensive health plan, 122–23; state department of mental health, 123; community mental health centers, 124; mayor's committees, 125; church groups, 125; special-interest groups, 126; United Fund, 126
—as volunteer, 126–27; advocacy service, 127; institutions and clinics, 128
Mental health centers. *See* Community mental health centers
Mental health clinics, 69–70; classification of, 70; licensing and accreditation of, 70; funding sources and sponsorship of, 71; private, 71; fees of, 71, 72, 76–77, 78; public, 72; teaching and research, 72–73; emer-

U.S. Government Printing Office, 113–14
U.S. Office of Education, 112
U.S. Social Security Administration, 114
U.S. Veterans Administration, 114

Vocational and interest tests, 34
Volunteer services. *See* Mental health activities

Walk-in clinics, 20, 43, 73–74, 98

X rays: skull, 30

Titles in the Series

MIGRANTS AND MALARIA IN AFRICA
R. Mansell Prothero

A PSYCHIATRIC RECORD MANUAL FOR THE HOSPITAL
Dorothy Smith Keller

RACISM AND MENTAL HEALTH
Essays
Charles V. Willie, Bernard M. Kramer, and Bertram S. Brown, Editors